HOW CAN YOU KNOW FOR SURE IF YOU OR SOMEONE IN YOUR FAMILY HAS A DRUG OR ALCOHOL PROBLEM?

ARE YOU TRAPPED IN THE DESTRUCTIVE PROCESS OF CODEPENDENCY?

WHAT DOES TOLERANCE HAVE TO DO WITH SOMEONE DEVELOPING A DRUG OR ALCOHOL PROBLEM?

COULD I BE ALCOHOLIC BECAUSE MY PARENTS WERE?

HOW DANGEROUS IS COCAINE?

These are but a few of the questions answered in *Growing Up Addicted*.

Readers praise *Growing Up Addicted*:

"For the first time I understood what I had been through. I wish I had read this years earlier in my recovery."

"I knew my family wasn't normal. Now I know why and what I can do about it."

"I read it, I cried, and I called my parents. Within two weeks I was in trea_____ _____ ____inning my own recovery."

GROWING UP ADDICTED

Why Our Children Abuse Alcohol and Drugs and What We Can Do About It

Stephen Arterburn

BALLANTINE BOOKS • NEW YORK

Grateful acknowledgment is made to the following for permission to reprint previously published material:

Marc B. Becker, Ph.D.: an excerpt from "Cocaine and the Workplace" by Marc B. Becker which appeared in the December 1985 issue of *The Messenger*, Vol. 1, No. 12. Reprinted by permission of Marc B. Becker, Ph.D., Chemical Dependency Treatment Specialist, Fullerton, Calif.

Fair Oaks Hospital: excerpt from "Cocaine Abuse Treatment" by Arnold M. Washton which appeared in the September 1985 issue of *Psychiatry Letter*, Vol. 3, Issue 9.

Library of Congress Catalog Card Number: 86-47848

ISBN 0-345-36114-8

Manufactured in the United States of America

First Ballantine/Epiphany Edition: May 1987
First Mass Market Edition: July 1989

This book is dedicated to my wife, Sandy. She is a most wonderful addiction.

A special thanks to all of the alcoholics and addicts I have had the pleasure of knowing over the years. Thank you for teaching me with your lives.

Contents

Contents

Introduction

It happens every day in thousands of homes. Unknowing, irresponsible parents help their children grow up addicted to alcohol and never consider the consequences. It might begin with adding a touch of booze to the formula to help quiet a child. It could occur from not intervening when the symptoms of addiction show up in the teen and post-teen years. There are many ways that parents can ensure that they have addicted their children

When mothers drink and drug while they are pregnant, their babies in the womb drink and drug also. Babies become addicted from alcohol and drugs passed through the bloodstream, mainlined into the unborn child. I attended a party where I observed a pregnant lady smoke and down one beer after another. I finally could not resist asking her if she was aware of the danger she was placing her child in. She told me that her physician had told her it was safe to drink two drinks a day. She had had nothing to drink all week, so she thought it was okay to combine the drinks from previous days into one evening. Stupidity or naïveté produces baby addicts and fetal alcohol syndrome in infants who become helpless victims before birth.

There is still another way that parents produce addicted children. ''For fun,'' they allow their preschoolers to have drugs or alcohol just to see the reaction. This form of child abuse sets the time clock of addiction in motion and almost guarantees a future alcoholic or drug addict. Other parents, sick parents, attempt to destroy their children by injecting them with heroin or teaching them to snort cocaine. These are extreme cases of abuse that lead to addiction. They are not the most common means by which parents addict or children grow up addicted. The other means by which children grow up addicted is what this book is all about. It is a book about addiction and how child addicts and alcoholics become teenage addicts and alcoholics who become adult addicts and alcoholics.

The bad news is that when teenagers drink and take drugs, they usually start by the time they are in the seventh grade. The good news is that parents, friends, and schools can keep even the high-risk kids clean. If a child is going to say no to alcohol or drugs, it will be because of the role of the parent. School drug education programs have little effect alone, but when combined with parental support and guidance, they can be effective. The parents are the biggest factor in the choice to drink or drug. This is not a book about drug use or the choice to drink. It is about addiction, a condition far more complicated and deadly than the choice to drink or use drugs.

There is a growing trend toward easy use of alcohol and drugs. This is indicative of the growing problem of addiction which we are experiencing now, and which will continue to increase if the addiction tide is not turnéd. There is evidence that more children are drinking and taking drugs at an earlier age. One study has revealed that over one third of all sixth graders have tried alcohol compared to only one tenth of all sixth graders just a few years ago. This is scary when you consider that the younger a child drinks, the faster the addiction clock ticks. The appeal for the youngster to drink is a strong force today. Spuds Mackenzie and the sweet taste of wine coolers are merely two enhancers of the urge for kids to start drinking younger. And younger drinkers make more addicts in later life.

Early alcohol use is coupled with the problem of campuses overflowing with drugs. Out of one group of one-hundred adolescents calling the hotline 1-800-COCAINE, fifty-seven said they bought their drugs in school, and eighty-two said their teachers were unaware that they use drugs.

"Easy availability of drugs in school is escalating the problem," says Dr. Mark S. Gold, founder of the help line and director of research at Fair Oaks Hospital in Summit, New Jersey.

Other reports confirm that the incidence of teenage drug abuse is increasing. A new report has led some experts to warn that a sociological time bomb may be ticking among the nation's high school students. A University of Michigan survey of new high school graduates showed drug abuse is on the increase. The most significant increase was in those who snort cocaine. One in eight said they had used cocaine over the past year. That was the highest figure in a decade. This is only part of the equation that makes the United States the highest drug user in the industrialized world.* A federal study revealed 617 cocaine deaths in 1984, up 77 percent in one year. Commenting on the problem, psychologist Lloyd Johnston of the University of Michigan cautioned that the United States may "see an already serious epidemic expand even further."

Because the problem is worsening, law enforcement, educators, and volunteers are increasing efforts to reduce the problem. When those efforts prove successful, drug and alcohol use will decrease and so will crime, right along with it. Recently the Justice Department did a spot testing of the correlation between drug abuse and criminal acts. Within a forty-eight-hour period, every person arrested for a non-domestic crime was tested for drugs in their system. The incidence was alarming. Over 70 percent of those tested, tested positive for an illegal drug. Because of these and similar statistics and the rapid spread of AIDS among intravenous drug users, there is a call to act. That call placed the national drug problem on the political agenda for the first time in 1988. The 1988 presidential election saw the war on drugs, the deterioration of the inner city due to drugs, and the rapid increase of urban drug problems as major campaign issues. Our nation's leaders have been called to act to reduce the escalation of drug use in America.

There is no question that early use, abuse, and addiction are on the increase. Hot lines, counselors, and treatment centers all attest to the growing addiction problem. You would have to bury your head in the sand to avoid the evidence of drug-related problems—or simply not care about the problem at all. But there are problems other than addiction associated with drug and alcohol use. Depression, suicide, overdose, dealing, theft, drunk driving, and family breakups all have their own consequences separate from the development of addiction.

The use of more than one chemical, called polydrug abuse, adds to a child's teenage depression. This deep depression is frequently linked to the rise in teenage suicide, which is up 150

*Monday Morning Report, vol. 12, no. 2 (25 January 1988). A Publication of Alcohol Research Information Services.

percent since 1950. That in itself is somewhat of an epidemic, at least a sickening phenomenon. The blue-ribbon committee that revealed the suicide statistics, the Business Advisory Commission of the Education Commission of the States, also found that 30 percent of adolescents had used an illegal drug in the past month and 37 percent had been involved in heavy drinking. It is important to note the reason why business and government leaders worry about our young people. They fear that due to the loss of kids through drugs or booze, there will be a shortage of skilled labor. They also know that without help, these kids cannot lead productive lives and contribute to society.

The statistical data vary from report to report as to how much alcohol and drug problems are on the increase, but they all point to an increase. There is no indication of a decline. As drug and alcohol use climb, so do the problems manifested from that use. Continuing to consider the link between alcohol and drugs and suicide, the evidence is staggering. Teens who commit suicide today are ten times more likely to be drunk or high on drugs than those who killed themselves twenty years ago. When intoxicated, suicidal youngsters are seven times more likely to use a gun to kill themselves. Dr. Dave Brent, University of Pittsburgh assistant child psychiatry professor, states, "Maybe one reason for the increase in teen suicide is the increase in drug and alcohol use." Drugs and alcohol kill. The saddest form of the destruction is when the effects of drugs and alcohol remove the will to live, and teenagers take their own lives.

Another major life threat from alcohol and drugs is driving while intoxicated. Alcohol-related crashes alone number in the tens of thousands. At least 65 percent of those in single-car crashes were legally drunk. For those ages fifteen to twenty-four, drunk driving is the number one killer. It is the reason that, while the life expectancy increases in all other age groups because of modern technology, it has gone down among the young. Every night drunk drivers drive a loaded pistol at us all, and every night there are explosions where alcohol and a driver produced death. Aside from driving, alcohol is involved in one out of every thirteen deaths; according to the National Academy of Science, 150,000 deaths a year involve alcohol. And remember, the trend is not getting better; it is getting worse.

Alcoholism and drug addiction are not problems unto themselves. Each is a way of life that produces results in many other areas. Addiction produces death through overdose. Every year two or three young movie stars are lost to overdose of some drug. Addiction also causes crime; people steal to buy alcohol and drugs. In addition, alcohol and drugs ruin families, breaking them up and taking a tremendous emotional toll. Nothing can so thoroughly destroy a life as alcohol and drugs.

The trend will be difficult to change. It is bred into the fabric of our society. No longer are home, school, and church the major influences to thousands of young people. Influence now comes from television, movies, music, and videos. These are void of traditional values. They often portray alcohol and drug use as part of growing up in America. They glamorize and popularize the most deadly tool our children can get their hands on.

How are we going to change all this? It certainly will not be easy. Change comes from a willingness to adjust attitudes first, then change actions or initiate action later. We must look through our old prejudices and search for truth. We must stop pointing a finger at each other—parents at teachers, teachers at parents—and each accept responsibility to do whatever is possible to curb this growing problem. It affects our young in epidemic proportions and produces adults who are scarred and traumatized by the effects of chemicals.

Everyone must see the need to increase organized, cooperative prevention efforts and participate in bringing government, schools, and families together to solve the problems *early*, not after years of addiction. Where there are no resources for treatment, resources are to be developed. When people finally decide to recover, the entire community must support that recovery. When everyone works together, when attitudes become constructive rather than judgmental, schools change, families change, and communities change. But the beginning is found at the heart of a new attitude.

Some still function under old attitudes. They believe the way to stop the problem is to scare the kids—yell at them, show them jails, and show them drug addicts. But this type of approach has minimal lasting value. What is so ironic about this approach is that it is indicative of the mentality of addiction. The scare tactic, just like the injection of heroin in a dark alley, is an attempt at a "quick fix." Sick societies, like sick people, are not fixed quickly. Only with new information and new attitudes can comprehensive programs be developed to prevent, treat, and support the recovery from drug and alcohol problems.

Growing Up Addicted can be a tool to begin to change attitudes. But if it is to do that, it must be read with an open mind and objectivity. Let me give you an example of how openness can change an attitude. There are a lot of folks who are scared about what illegal drugs are doing to kids. They want to stamp out these drugs, bring in the troops, and eradicate them from the face of the earth. Well, that is a nice idea. It would not hurt one bit. But look at what that approach does. It focuses all the attention on what *we* can do to *them*. It identifies the illegal stuff as the enemy. And it appoints the military and law enforcement as the ones to change society. There is another way to approach the problem.

To be effective, stopping people from growing up addicted begins when adults take care of their own problems. When they quit trying to fix kids and start fixing themselves, society—kids and all—begins to recover. Rather than focus on the illegal stuff, which is more glamorous and dramatic, we need to completely understand the stuff you buy at a grocery store down the street. The stuff down at the store ends up in cabinets and on counters at home. It becomes a part of a life-style. It is consumed by far more than will ever do heroin, cocaine, or marijuana. It is just not as interesting as the other. And for many, objectivity about alcohol is lost because it hits too close to home.

Now, do not get the wrong idea. As you read further, you will discover that I am no neo-prohibitionist. Please keep the objectivity through to the end. But let me present an example of what I am explaining. *Time* had a recent article on the drug "crack," distributed in small, pellet-size "rocks" on the streets of New York. People are intrigued to know that it sells for only ten dollars for a small plastic vial. The effects are instantaneous and intense. The rush from smoking it rather than snorting it has made it the drug of the moment. *Time* reported: "Drug addicts are always looking for the ultimate high, and they all agree that crack is the ultimate. The addiction rate is fast and high, and the low price is alluring." As informative as that is, and as interesting, does it help the problem? Everyone wants to read about the new stuff the kids are doing on the streets of New York, but they are not nearly as interested in taking action at home.

More kids will spend ten dollars on a case of beer than they will on a hit of crack. More families will be destroyed from alcoholism than heroin. More jobs will be lost to alcohol than to marijuana. So if we are to solve the problem, we cannot simply increase our knowledge of illegal street drugs; we must learn about the accepted chemicals that are legal. While perhaps 20 to 30 percent of our high school seniors will use an illegal substance, and we regret the percentage is growing, it is far more important to focus on the 98 percent who will drink and the 20 to 30 percent who will become alcoholic.

Most people do not need more information on illegal drugs. You take them, you develop a tolerance, become addicted, spend a lot of money, and wind up miserable. The signs and symptoms are obvious early on, and the behavioral changes are quite marked. The last portion of this book covers drugs for those who have a complete lack of awareness about them, but it is not nearly as important as the material on alcoholism. Attitudes about alcoholism have a long way to go before real change can take place. Adults must deal with their problems first; then they will successfully help kids with drug and alcohol problems.

What is there to learn about alcoholism? What can be said that has not been repeated many times? A lot. For instance, alcoholism is invisible in its early symptoms, while drug addiction is quite obvious. While drinking, including problem drinking, can be learned, alcoholism cannot. Taking drugs is a behavior; addiction is not. Drinking is a behavior; alcoholism is a disease. If you find yourself disagreeing, you are not alone. A lot of these concepts fly in the face of long-held beliefs about drinking and drunkenness. To add fuel to the fire, did you know that drunkenness is not necessarily a symptom of alcoholism? If that last statement was enough to really irritate you, I hope you will read on. There is plenty of evidence to substantiate the claim.

Did you realize that 35 percent of everyone in a general hospital suffer from alcoholism or alcohol-related problems? Or that in psychiatric and orthopedic wards, the rate goes to 50 percent? Most of those people will never be diagnosed as alcoholics. They will go through life breaking limbs, destroying livers, and separating families, but they will never have a diagnosis of alcoholism. Many physicians simply are unwilling to use that label or are unaware of how prevalent the problem is. It points up how badly we need to examine alcoholism. It is an old problem that too few are doing too little about.

Back in 1956, the American Medical Association declared that alcoholism is a disease. It outlined the signs and symptoms that led to a diagnosis of alcoholism. But the unique symptoms that form alcoholism were identified as a special problem long before the AMA's position. Dr. Benjamin Rush, a signer of the Declaration of Independence, was also this country's first psychiatrist. He wrote of alcoholism as something different from social drinking or even occasional intoxication. Research into the problem has come a long way since then, but it confirms Rush's basic idea.

In recent years, most of the research about alcoholism has centered on the genetic and hereditary aspects of alcoholism. Because of this new understanding, the problem is being completely redefined. The myth that alcoholics are drunk all the time is giving way to the recognition that many alcoholics remain undiscovered, working and living outwardly normal lives, until an alcohol-related disease or accident suddenly cuts them down. The myth that alcoholism is always psychologically caused is giving way to a realization that it is in large measure biologically determined. Drinking is a choice; alcoholism is not. The hope is that this new evidence can allow the problem to be identified earlier so that a lot of waste is prevented.

Much of this book focuses on the controversial evidence of the genetic predisposition to alcoholism, because in that focus there is hope. A new way of thinking, a new attitude toward alcoholism, will allow millions more to recover. Now too few do. It is my desire that the physiological emphasis will not scare you away. Nothing but facts and truth are presented. But in addition to the predisposition focus, there is material designed to give you a true understanding of the emotional trauma experienced by the alcoholic. This enables some to help alcoholics better and others to recognize alcoholism within themselves.

If somehow we as adults can solve our alcohol and drug problems first, I believe we can finally help our kids with theirs. If we can stop pointing fingers and start taking action, we will triumph over addiction. We will identify problems sooner and initiate treatment more quickly. We will build a peer pressure base that will allow a "no" in the face of alcohol and drugs rather than a forced "yes." It is to that end that *Growing Up Addicted* is written.

CHAPTER ONE

STEPHANIE: THE BEGINNING

Twelve years ago, I was working at an alcoholism treatment center in Texas. It was my first job in the field of addiction as an alcoholism counselor. One Saturday morning, having finished lecturing to a group of patients and their families, I went into my office to chart in the medical records the participation of the patients. While I was charting, the head nurse buzzed me on the intercom and told me that someone was on the phone inquiring about the treatment center. I told her I would take the call, and I punched the flashing button to speak with the inquirer.

"Hello. How can I help you?" I asked.

Very softly and with a cracking voice, the man on the other end replied, "I need to know about your program."

"What is the problem?" I asked.

"It's my daughter. I think she has a problem with alcohol. I want to know what kind of help is available."

I took some information from him, his address, phone number, and other details. I then asked him to bring his daughter down to the hospital. He agreed and said that he and his wife would bring her in about an hour. I assured him that I would wait until they arrived and that he had done the right thing in calling.

At about four o'clock I met the Westmorelands (not their real name) in the lobby and escorted them back to my office. Their sixteen-year-old daughter, Stephanie, was very attractive, had long blond hair, and was staring at the floor. It was not until she sat down in my office that I saw what she was trying to hide. I no longer wondered why Mr. Westmoreland had called. Stephanie's face was black and blue from what appeared to be a severe beating. Her left eye was without any white, only bright red from broken blood vessels. She hung her head and cried throughout the session.

What I was seeing disturbed me terribly. I suspected child abuse and had no experience in how to handle the situation legally. I could think of no other explanation than that her father had beaten her while he or she or both were intoxicated. Family violence was quite common in the homes where alcoholism progressed.

I also lacked experience in dealing with adolescents. All of our patients were adults. But in spite of my caution, I knew that I must proceed decisively. If the family suspected that I was overwhelmed by the situation, they would not allow me to help, and they might not seek help again for a very long time—if ever. I wanted to help, so I began gathering information. The unfolding story was my first real-life encounter with adolescent alcoholism. It was similar to many other stories I would hear over the years to come. Although each story would have different details and different localities, it would share some of the same elements as the Westmoreland story. Someone in the family would have an alcohol problem, the family would try to help, but the problem would progress. Finally, after some crisis, help would be sought. The crisis for Stephanie Westmoreland led her father to call for help. And with that call hope became a reality for the first time in six years of progressing alcoholism. The following three chapters are Stephanie's story.

Stephanie's father, Thomas Westmoreland, was a forty-one-year-old rancher who lived a few miles outside of Fort Worth. A self-assured man, he tasted affluence in his late thirties when Texaco discovered oil in his back pasture. He eventually quit his job as a construction foreman for Brown and Root Construction Company and attempted to expand his wealth through raising and selling Arabian horses. His venture had proven to be very successful.

Thomas was a tall, muscular man who appeared to possess great physical strength. His father, who had been a rancher, died of liver disease after years of heavy drinking. Thomas had sold some of the land left by his father in order to pay for four years of college at Texas A&M University in College Station. His animal husbandry degree had come in handy in horse ranching.

Thomas, like his father, was a heavy drinker. He had begun

drinking when in high school and had rarely gone a day without a drink since then. He was rarely drunk, even though he might drink a couple of six-packs of beer in one evening watching television. His tolerance was very high.

He never drank during the day, and although in earlier years he had liked to "drink with the boys," most of his drinking over the past few years had been at home. He worked hard and felt that the alcohol was harmless, relaxing. His love for beer, he said, was strictly a matter of taste.

Thomas loved his wife and he loved his children. He was not extremely affectionate, but he had no trouble in expressing his love to his family. In the past few years he had grown increasingly moody, for unexplainable reasons. His moods would vacillate between extreme joy and exhilaration and the depths of depression. He would go for days in a tearful state, only to wind up cheerful and in a "great mood" for no apparent reason. He had begun to explain the condition to me by saying that he had "kinda' lost control of my emotions lately."

It was apparent from our conversation that he cared very deeply about Stephanie. He was concerned and afraid of what might happen if she did not stop drinking. He was embarrassed to have called, but he could think of no alternative. He had become desperate in his desire to help Stephanie.

Cynthia Westmoreland was thirty-seven years old but looked five years younger. She had married Thomas when she was eighteen years old, three days after high school graduation. Raised in a very strict Southern Baptist home, her family values stayed with her into adulthood. She never drank or smoked and each Sunday, with or without Thomas, she would drive into Fort Worth to attend services at College Avenue Baptist Church.

Cynthia had always loved her husband very much, but she never loved his drinking. It had always been the one thing about Thomas that she wanted to change. She believed what her parents had taught her, that alcohol was an evil substance, and no good would ever come from its consumption. When Thomas would come home with alcohol on his breath, she would never say a word about it. She would just quote the pastor's wife: "It's my job to love my husband; it's God's job to make him good." But deep inside her, anger over the alcohol had increased with the years of drinking. It also embarrassed her at the church because everyone knew that Thomas loved to drink.

Cynthia loved her children very much. She had been actively involved in all their activities, from baseball and soccer to the youth choir at church. She had even played the piano for the choir while Stephanie was a member. Being so involved in her children's lives, watching them grow up from such a close vantage point, she never imagined that alcohol would ever be a problem. That her daughter was an adolescent alcoholic was a nightmare that she had never dreamed.

Shortly after their marriage, Thomas and Cynthia had their first child, a boy they named Stansell. Stansell was now, at seventeen, a "model child"—not only according to Thomas and Cynthia, but to everyone else who knew Stansell and the Westmoreland family. He was loved by almost everyone, except those who were jealous of his many talents and rare integrity.

Stansell played fullback on the district championship football team. He had obtained a scholarship to attend Texas A&M, just like his father. But his major would not be animal husbandry. His field of study would be architecture. Of all of Stansell's talents, perhaps his greatest was what he could conceptualize, design, and transfer to paper. He had already translated that talent into a car and a big savings account. By drawing for a landscape architectural firm, he had been able to buy the car of his dreams, a 1957 red-and-white Chevrolet Corvette. With his grades and talents, he could have attended college on scholarship anywhere he wanted. But he felt driven to make his father proud of him, and he believed that that pride would be felt only for a star performance at Texas A&M University.

Boys like Stansell are rare. He was skilled, confident, and the rock of emotional stability to everyone he met. He was determined to achieve and determined to be successful. And he would not allow anything to stand in the way of his quest for that success. So, very early on, he had vowed never to use any drugs or drink any alcohol. He had kept that commitment except for one occasion.

On Thomas's fortieth birthday, he asked Stansell to lead the guests in a "real" toast. Reluctant at first, Stansell took his first drink at the age of sixteen in a crowd of his parents' friends. But although his mind accepted his father's request, his body said a very violent no to the large post-toast gulp; the planned tribute to his father terminated with Stansell spewing the "bubbly" on both his father and mother. The incident disturbed Stansell, but those at the party felt it was only a proof of the naïve nature of a very gentle young man.

Stansell absolutely worshipped Stephanie. He felt his sister was the most special girl in the world. He had, at a young age, appointed himself Stephanie's protector and chief adviser. There was nothing that he would not do for his little sister. He had gone so far as to have a little pre-date chat with everyone she had gone out with. His lecture included guidelines for proper conduct, as well as a time for questions when the agenda of the date was presented. Each session ended with the threat of a slow and painful death if anything happened to his sister.

It was odd that Stansell adored his sister so much but had little time or interest for other girls. He viewed them as a potential threat to his ultimate success. His belief was that he would do best to achieve and accomplish now; once he had made it, there would be plenty of time for relationships. Early marriage was no option for Stansell.

Other than his lack of girlfriends, Stansell appeared to be the All-American boy and more. His parents felt that he would do all that he planned in his life, and that his example was a good one for the two girls. Stephanie and her younger sister, Stella, did admire their older brother, but they both knew he was a tough act to follow. While he was making headlines, they had a difficult time establishing their own identity as other than Stansell's little sisters.

Stella's name was determined in part by the Westmorelands' desire to have all the children's names begin with the letter S. Stella was twelve years old. She looked up to her brother but idolized her sister. She would do anything for Stephanie and was totally dedicated to her well-being. Stella's dedication was not unusual for her age, but because of Stephanie's problem with alcohol, that dedication was often stretched beyond normal.

One weekend, six months before my meeting the Westmorelands, they had left town to spend the weekend alone. It was a weekend they had promised themselves for years. They left the kids to take care of themselves, with promises that they would all stay together, so they were not really worried.

The first night that the parents were away, Stephanie sneaked out the window at midnight to meet one of her friends and drink. Stella heard the car drive up in front, and she heard the window in her sister's room open as Stephanie climbed out and ran to the car. As the pair drove off, Stella lay in bed and cried. She loved her sister, and she knew what was going to happen. She had heard Stephanie return drunk early in the morning several times before.

Two hours later, Stella awoke to the sound of a car door slamming in front of the house. She heard the stumbling, shuffling feet of her sister as she drunkenly crossed the lawn back to her bedroom window. Then Stella heard the branches of a bush snap and the sudden rustling of the leaves as Stephanie fell below her window. Stella jumped out of bed, raced outside, and found her sister passed out under the window, lying in the bushes and flowers.

Stella began to cry as she walked back into her room. Once there, she grabbed two pillows and the covers from her bed. She rolled them into a bundle and returned outside to where Stephanie lay. Weeping and sobbing, she placed Stephanie's head on one of the pillows, covered her with the blankets from her bed, and lay down beside her. There she stayed, by Stephanie's side, crying herself to sleep, then waking and pleading with God not to let her sister die.

The next morning Stephanie woke up with no idea how she had ended up in the bushes. Stella reminded her of her late-night spree. Stephanie quickly realized what had happened and how her little sister had responded. She began to sob deeply, hugging and hanging on to Stella, promising her that she would never, never do it again, and begging Stella not to tell her parents. Stella knew it would be only a matter of time before the drama, in some similar form, was played out once again. She felt responsible to help Stephanie and protect her the best way she knew how. It was an awfully big task for a twelve-year-old girl, but she shouldered that task because she loved her older sister so much. That love, so openly demonstrated, only made Stephanie's guilt increase. And rather than motivating her to stop drinking, it led her to drink more and more.

Stephanie had her first drink when she was ten years old. This bright and beautiful little girl had spent the night with her best friend, Linda Jacobsen. She and three others her age fell victim to the connivings of Linda's brother. He concocted a special punch for the girls and persuaded each one to drink it.

For Stephanie, that first drink was a very fun experience. It made her feel warm all over, seconds after swallowing it. And then, just minutes later, she and her friends were all laughing and giggling and having the time of their lives. Soon they all wound down to a long night of sleep. The next morning, for all her fun, Stephanie paid the price of a severe headache and a sick stomach.

Morning-after queasiness was not enough to destroy Stephanie's desire to drink again; hung over as they were, she and Linda talked about their next drinking event. They determined that the safest way to ensure the supply was to meet some needs of Linda's older brother. They washed his car, cleaned his room, and did little errands so that he would help them acquire alcohol on the weekends. This continued for several years. She loved to drink with Linda, and rarely did they allow anyone to join their private parties. But at fourteen, Stephanie was allowed to date. When she entered the dating world, her supply sources changed, as did the experience of drinking.

Stephanie's beauty attracted many pursuers from the first day she was allowed to date. When she arrived at the Junior-Senior prom with her first suitor, the other guys knew that the dating game had a new entrant. Her arrival at that major function was as dramatic as a presentation at a debutante ball. The phone at her house began to ring relentlessly. She loved picking and choosing who would accompany her where. She quickly gravitated toward the "wild bunch" at school; she viewed the All-American types as boring. But her choices did not correspond with her parents' at all. She and her parents frequently argued about her dates. From those arguments, Stephanie learned a lesson she would never forget: she could do whatever she wanted, even if her parents did not approve. They simply would not tell her no. For Stephanie, there were no limitations other than the ones she placed on herself. At the age of fourteen, these were very few.

With the onset of her dating life came a new problem that surfaced every six weeks. Stephanie's freshman grades began to deteriorate. She was very bright and had always made A's, but those A's became mixed with some B's. Then the A's disappeared, and C's crept among the B's. Her grades deeply disappointed her parents and puzzled her teachers. Stephanie heard the pleadings from her teachers and from her parents, but they did not faze her at all. Her goals had been transformed in a very short time. She declined from wanting to do her very best to doing just enough to get by. She was so intelligent that she did not have to study at all to make C's and an occasional B. So she stopped studying and used that time to be with her friends.

The gradual descent of her grades was the first sign that a problem was developing. It was obvious on her second ninth-grade report card that the trend was downward. The grades had deteriorated because her discipline, her study habits, and her goals had all deteriorated. Her friends were not of the highest caliber, either. As her popularity decreased at school, her dependence on the more deviant kids increased. All her spare time was spent with them, so that the time with her family was almost nonexistent. Nor did she have time for extracurricular activities at school. Most of her nonclassroom hours were spent with her friends and in drinking. To Stephanie, they were all that mattered.

That first drink with Linda had made Stephanie feel good. The alcohol produced a warm feeling inside of her. And when she had consumed just enough, her mind would shift into a different gear. The "buzz" from the alcohol was more of a feeling of security to her. Her early drinking episodes, at ages ten, eleven, or twelve, had produced no obvious, identifiable problems, but now anyone looking at her grades, friends, and lack of involvement in school activities could see that all was not progressing normally for Stephanie.

What was progressing normally was her alcoholism. In its earliest stage there was no evidence that it existed, at least no evidence that parents or teachers could detect. The only thing different about her was *that* she drank and *how* she drank. But she hid her drinking from all but a very few. If someone could have seen how she drank at such a young age, the abnormality would have been apparent. Even at age eleven and twelve she was starting to develop a tolerance for alcohol that Linda and many others were not developing. At thirteen, when others would stop drinking after two or three beers, Stephanie would continue until she had drunk six or seven—and was less intoxicated and less affected by the alcohol than those who had drunk only two or three. If you did not notice that difference, you would not have known that anything was wrong.

The middle stage of her alcoholism developed as she started dating and drinking more frequently. The friends, the grades, and her disassociation from the family all indicated the development of a problem. But without knowing Stephanie drank, her parents never thought that alcohol had a part in her problems. They were convinced that it was a temporary phase. They believed that their beautiful daughter would pass through it and move into a more acceptable academic and social life. But the longer she stayed in this phase, the more obvious it was that emergence from it was not going to happen naturally.

It was hard for Stephanie's mother to realize that she was not just going through a normal developmental process. Out of desperation, Cynthia turned to her pastor for help. She told him about Stephanie's grades, her wild friends, and her change of attitude over the past couple of years. He had noticed that over the past six months Stephanie had stopped going to church, and he was concerned. He told Cynthia that Stephanie's only hope was to return to church, repent of her past sins, and renew her relationship with God. He felt that anything short of a total conversion would bring only temporary results. What was needed, he explained, was an eternal solution. He recommended that Cynthia have the fifteen-year-old come and see him.

Cynthia discussed the meeting with Thomas the next day. At first he was upset that the pastor had been consulted on this family matter but then realized it was better than doing nothing—and the time had clearly come for something to be done. They agreed that Stephanie would never accompany them to the pastor's office, so they planned to invite Reverend Owens over for dinner. Then, as the table was being cleared and the dishes washed, he could talk to Stephanie alone.

Two weeks later, Reverend Owens came to dinner. Stephanie was polite to the pastor but never looked at him or talked to him. Throughout dinner, the pastor praised the family for such things as Cynthia's involvement in the church and Stansell's outstanding accomplishments in school and sports. When dinner was over, as planned, Thomas and Cynthia began cleaning up and Reverend Owens asked Stephanie to step into the living room with him for a little talk.

After telling him that some friends were picking her up in a few minutes, Stephanie reluctantly agreed to give the pastor some time. Reverend Owens explained to her how much he cared about her as a person. He told her that he wanted the best for her in every way. He went on to describe the love and concern that her parents had for her. He mentioned all the wonderful blessings she had been given, such as her beauty, her nice home, and her wonderful family. Then he talked about God's love for her and how it was so much greater than his or her parents', and how all that she had been given by her parents had really been given to her by God through them. Reverend Owens explained that not only had God blessed her greatly, but that He would continue to bless her life in ways that she could not imagine. In exchange, God wanted only one thing—Stephanie's life. He told her that it was really quite a good bargain: if you give God you, God gives you everything. He chuckled as he said that it doesn't seem like God gets a very good deal in most cases.

Stephanie listened as he explained what God wanted for her. She began to cry, at first softly, but then loudly. She ran to her mother and hugged her, telling her how sorry she was and how she wanted to do better, that she wanted to change. She hugged her father and asked him to forgive her. He said that he would and that he loved her very much.

Reverend Owens asked Stephanie, Cynthia, and Thomas to join him in the living room, and they all bowed their heads as the pastor prayed. While he prayed, Stephanie and Cynthia, arms around each other, sobbed deeply. The pastor encouraged the family to pray together every night and to be sure and see him on Sunday after the church service. He would want to know how everything was going. With that invitation, he left the Westmorelands, feeling that his mission had been accomplished.

When Stephanie's friends came by, she told them she did not want to go out, so they left. Stephanie and her mother talked for a while, and then Stephanie went to her room to cry herself to sleep. Something had happened that night, and everyone hoped that it was the beginning of a totally new life for Stephanie. Stephanie wanted a new way of life. She felt trapped in her lifestyle. She realized that she had left so much behind to achieve so little. She felt that she had taken her first steps into change and was aware of a tremendous feeling of relief. She felt very clean that night.

Throughout the evening, there had been no mention of alcohol. Reverend Owens certainly had not talked about it; he did not even know that Stephanie was a drinker. Cynthia and Thomas knew that Stephanie had been drinking from time to time, but they never even considered that as part of the problem.

And Stephanie, at the moment of greatest remorse, did not confess her infatuation with alcohol or her drinking behavior. So the Westmorelands, with new hopes and dreams for their fifteen-year-old daughter, still had no idea that Stephanie was an alcoholic. To them, she had been in a bad phase. With the help of Reverend Owens, that phase was over. They believed that Stephanie, the Stephanie they loved so much, was back. They prayed that she was back for good.

Over the next few days, Stephanie was determined to make the necessary changes to clean up her act. She told herself that she would never drink again. She went so far as to promise that she would not go out with anyone who drank or took drugs. She told her mother she wanted to go to church with her every Sunday. And she promised that her primary goal would be to improve her grades and keep them up. With a whole new perspective on life, Stephanie realized that she had a problem with alcohol—although she never told anyone—and she believed that she could live without it. She wanted to recapture some of what she had lost over the past few years. She also wanted to make up for some of the problems she had caused for her family. The youngest member of the family, Stella, needed a good example to follow. Stephanie wanted to be the model big sister.

Over the next couple of weeks, Stephanie's attitude changed dramatically. She did not spend after-school time with her old friends, but in studying and reading. Her parents could not have been more pleased with what they saw. It was as if a miracle had occurred. Their hopes and dreams had been fulfilled and their prayers answered. They believed that once again they could experience life as a normal family. Whatever the problem was, they all believed that it was over. Their little Stephanie was a beautiful person and a daughter they could be proud of.

CHAPTER TWO

STEPHANIE: THE PROGRESSION

Family outings and church activities filled the summer months following Stephanie's decision to change. Stephanie returned to the church choir and made new friends there. Her mother played the piano and enjoyed every minute of those times together. Reverend Owens was delighted to see active participation by the whole family, including Thomas. He felt that his visit had been instrumental in the complete turnaround of Stephanie's life. When I talked to him later, he regretted that he had not understood the full extent of the problem.

The greatest event of that summer for Stephanie was turning sixteen, because she could legally drive into town. The family celebrated her sixteenth birthday at the Old Swiss House. When it was time for dessert, the waiter carried in a huge cake with sixteen candles—and nestled in the middle of the cake was a set of car keys. She blew out the candles and picked up the keys, and her father ushered her out the door. Parked at the entrance of the restaurant, wrapped in a big red bow, was a pink Volkswagen "bug" with a white convertible top. It was the happiest day of Stephanie's life.

School started not long after that. Stephanie did very well the first six weeks, making all A's except for one B. She had studied hard and earned her grades. She was able to prove to her parents that the car would not stand in her way of achieving to the best of her ability, and she continued to involve herself in church. From every angle it appeared that Stephanie had solved her problems. But that appearance changed drastically on a Saturday night in November.

Thomas picked up the phone at 11:45 P.M. to hear the stern voice of a police officer on the other end. She informed Thomas that his daughter had been picked up about 10:30 after another officer had spotted her driving erratically in downtown Fort Worth. She had been booked on charges of driving while intoxicated. The officer told Thomas that he could post bail and take Stephanie home. Stunned and shocked, he broke the news to his wife and went down to the police station. He took Stansell along to drive Stephanie's car home.

On the way to the station, Thomas asked Stansell what he knew about Stephanie's drinking habits. Stansell said that he was sure she had drunk alcohol in the past but that he did not know of any problem. He told his father he thought all that was behind Stephanie. As fas as he knew, she had not been drinking at all that summer. But Stansell was not totally truthful. He knew, but didn't say, that during the last school year, Stephanie had developed a reputation as a heavy drinker. It was a reputation that hurt Stansell very much.

When they arrived, Stephanie was in tears. Thomas paid the money and left with Stephanie. The parents of the two girls riding with Stephanie had already picked them up. Once in the car, Stephanie explained what had happened. Her version of the evening was similar to her first drinking experience. She claimed that they had gone to a party at one of their friends' homes, where one of the boys had put some "ever-clear" liquor in the punch. She said she had no idea that she was drinking alcohol until it was too late. She did not think she was drunk, so she started to take her friends home. On her way, the police officer pulled her over, gave her a couple of tests for intoxication, and took her to the police station.

Thomas believed his daughter, at least the part about not knowing the alcohol was in the punch. He certainly did not see this as an indicator of an alcohol problem. What he could not tolerate was the fact that once she did drink, she drove the car. As a result, he did something he had never done before. He took the car away and grounded her for six weeks. Stephanie thought she had gotten off pretty easily, especially when she discovered that her father's attorney was able to have all the charges dismissed. Her record was clean.

Thomas and Cynthia were embarrassed by the whole episode. They had to do quite a bit of explaining as rumors about the incident spread. But the embarrassment quickly passed, as did the six weeks of grounding for Stephanie. When they were over, her freedom was restored and her car returned. But Stephanie's attitude was not restored. As her punishment had continued, her anger had increased. But the most overwhelming thing was her intense guilt. The events of the evening of her drunk driving were not as she had explained. What appeared to be the innocent act of an adolescent was actually the result of a predictable return to the use of alcohol, her chemical addiction.

Stephanie had suffered a classical relapse. She had returned to drinking as a result of compromising some of the commitments she made before summer. The biggest compromise was in the area of relationships. She had made the commitment not to date people who drank or took drugs. When she broke that commitment, she took her first step back into addiction. She broke the commitment when a very handsome, popular boy from her church took her out on a date. On their first date he asked her if she would like for him to obtain some alcohol. She said no and expressed surprise that he drank at all. But she did not refuse to see him again. On their third date, he brought tequila, ice, and all the mixers needed to make margaritas. And even though she did not drink, he did, along with the couple they brought with them. She wanted to continue seeing him. It was only a matter of time before she was drinking again. The compromise was the key element in her relapse into drinking. And once the drinking started again, the rest of her life began to fall apart. She did well in covering up the problems until the drunk driving charge. She was even able to cover up what truly happened that night.

That night was no different from the past few weekend nights. She and her friends met some boys, who always brought the alcohol, and went to a park close to the Trinity River. There they would drink, get drunk, often become involved sexually, then go home. For some of the kids the drinking ended as they said good-bye. But for Stephanie, it did not. She was obsessed with the stuff. She would spend hours thinking about her next drink, how she would get it and how she would cover up the drinking. Most of her drinking was done alone, except for those weekend gatherings at the park.

Although Stephanie was drinking almost daily, she was rarely drunk. She had such a high tolerance for the chemical that two six-packs of beer would not intoxicate her at all. She would often sneak away at noon and have what she called ''liquid lunches'' of vodka and orange juice. But none of her teachers suspected that she drank, because she showed no apparent signs of intoxication. Her tolerance protected her from discovery. It also trapped her more deeply into a physical addiction every day that she drank.

Although there were no outward signs of intoxication, many indicators started to surface that pointed toward a renewal of her problems. Her schoolwork once again began to decline drastically. She no longer spent time studying or reading. Most of her time was spent with the old friends who had arrived back on the scene. She also stopped her church involvement. Stephanie wanted no part of it or of the Reverend Owens. Her attitude change was extreme. Although her parents did not know what was wrong, they knew that *something* was. The "phase" she had been in before had returned, and Stephanie appeared to be in it deeper than ever.

Cynthia was very disturbed at seeing her daughter change so dramatically in such a short time. She was not the only one who was deeply concerned. Mrs. Cummings, Stephanie's English teacher, phoned Cynthia to discuss Stephanie's recent poor performance and the undesirable relationships she was establishing. Cynthia could not deny that something was wrong and asked for a suggestion on how to handle the problem. Mrs. Cummings suggested that it was obviously a behavioral problem and that behavior could be changed through rewards and punishment. She pointed out that the rewards of good grades, a car, and freedom had not produced the desired changes, so that punishment was the only alternative. She told Cynthia that she and Thomas must be more strict. Stephanie needed to be brought into submission.

With that advice, Cynthia developed a plan with Thomas to motivate Stephanie to change. They gave her a curfew, limited her use of the car, and forced her to study two hours every evening. They also demanded that one weekend night, rather than going out, her friends must come to the Westmorelands'. Stephanie fell into angry compliance, but her sneaking out at night increased, as did her drinking to the point of drunkenness. Her anger grew as her parents set more restrictions and laid out more difficult rules. After a couple of weeks, the household was a living hell, full of turmoil. The Westmorelands felt that they had made a terrible mistake.

One evening, after a terrible argument at dinner, Stephanie waited for everyone to go to sleep and then drank half of a fifth of vodka she had hidden in her room. She gulped it hard and fast and straight, then passed out. The next morning Cynthia went in to wake her for school and found the empty vodka bottle on the floor and Stephanie in very bad shape. The moment her mother woke her, Stephanie threw up and began shaking. She told her mother that the bottle had only contained a small amount and she had brought it home just to see what it tasted like, that she thought it would be safer to drink at home alone rather than with the other kids . . . that she did not want to get arrested again.

Cynthia, troubled, drove Stephanie to the family physician's office rather than to school. The doctor talked to Mrs. Westmoreland alone before seeing Stephanie. Cynthia described what had been happening over the past few weeks. The physician met with Stephanie for about half an hour, then saw Cynthia alone.

He told her that he believed Stephanie was having an adolescent adjustment reaction, that she was actually afraid of growing up. Allowing the vodka bottle to be found was Stephanie's way of crying out for help; he told Cynthia that he was no psychiatrist but had seen this happen frequently over the years. He suggested that both Thomas and Cynthia let up on Stephanie, give her some room to breathe and encourage her as she tried to find her way toward adulthood. He prescribed Valium and told her to give the pills to Stephanie for the next couple of weeks until things settled down a little for her.

Once at home, Cynthia put Stephanie to bed and gave her a Valium to help her relax. It was the first time Stephanie had ever taken a mood-altering chemical other than alcohol. The physician and her mother had introduced her to a neat and tidy way of feeling better, and Stephanie sought to feel that way often. She drank much less and became dependent on the availability of the Valium three times a day. For a while, she was satisfied with her new chemical friend.

When the pharmacist asked him for a third refill of the Valium the doctor phoned Cynthia. She told him that Stephanie had been more subdued and less angry since their visit and was doing much better. There had been no evidence of drinking. After hearing her describe Stephanie's behavior, the physician suggested that Mrs. Westmoreland take Stephanie to see a psychologist. He would continue to prescribe Valium if she would put Stephanie into therapy with a specialist in adolescent psychology.

Thomas was furious when he found out that his daughter had an appointment with a psychologist. He did not believe in "shrinks" of any kind. He felt that his family problems were not the business of someone who "probably never had any kids anyway." But he consented when Cynthia told him that even Reverend Owens considered it the only alternative. Nothing else had worked, and Stephanie was not getting better. Since she had seen their physician, Stephanie appeared better, but Cynthia had to admit that progress was not being made.

A week later Stephanie and her mother went to see an adolescent psychologist in Arlington, Texas. The psychologist met with mother and daughter together for the first session. Stephanie was quiet most of the time as her mother expressed her concerns about Stephanie's friends, grades, attitude, and the fact that she was continuing to take medication. Cynthia also briefly described the two events that involved alcohol and her disappointment in learning that Stephanie drank. She had hoped that Stephanie and her other two children would have developed a life-style devoid of alcohol.

Cynthia also described the miraculous change Stephanie had made after the visit from Reverend Owens. She talked of what a great few months it had been for Stephanie and the whole family, and how confused and hurt she had become when Stephanie returned to her old life-style. She desperately needed some answers, she said, and some results.

The psychologist asked Stephanie how she felt about what her mother had said. She was quiet and unresponsive but did eventually say that she was "different" and that her parents did not understand. At the end of the session, it was agreed that Stephanie would return for at least eight weeks. Cynthia left the office with a sense of hope. She had liked the psychologist and felt that he could be trusted to help Stephanie and the family.

The following day, the psychologist phoned Cynthia to discuss her daughter. He told her that he felt Stephanie was experiencing a deep depression and that all the problem behavior was a vain attempt by Stephanie to cope with it. Once the depression lifted, Stephanie would not need to drink, and her attitude would improve as her mood lifted. He told Cynthia he was calling the family physician and would recommend that the Valium prescription be replaced with an antidepressant or mood-elevating drug known as Triavil, which he said should assist the therapeutic process. The tablets would only be temporary, until he was able to probe into Stephanie to discover the root of all her problems.

Over the next few weeks, Stephanie's mood lightened and she was not as depressed as before. Her parents were encouraged by what they saw as real progress. The psychologist seemed to know what he was doing, and Stephanie seemed once again on the road to recovery.

It was not long before that opinion changed completely. The change came the day before Thomas Westmoreland called the hospital. It was the last crisis that finally led to Thomas taking responsibility for finding help for Stephanie. Until then he had left most of the decisions concerning Stephanie to his wife, but because of what happened that Friday, Thomas was ready and willing to do whatever it took to save his daughter.

That Friday night had started off innocently enough. The family had dinner together, and then Stansell announced that a friend was coming by to pick him up and they were going to the show together. When he went to his room to dress for his outing, Stephanie followed him. She asked if he would let her and her friend drive his beloved classic Corvette into Fort Worth to get a Coke and come home. She promised that they would not be gone over two hours and that there would be no alcohol. Stansell loved his car, but he loved his sister much more. Although he felt very awkward about it, he simply could not refuse Stephanie's request. She was thrilled and hurried to get ready; by seven she was racing out the door yelling that she would return by nine o'clock. Stansell ran after her and gave her one final warning to be careful, no booze, and be back by nine.

Stephanie picked up her friend Julie, and they set out for a hangout just east of the Ridgemar Mall, where they met some other friends and talked for a few minutes. Then they left to drive around in Stansell's car. They had been riding around for about ten minutes when they stopped at a red light. As they waited for the light to change, two boys in a black Porsche pulled up beside them and yelled out that they liked the car. Stephanie and Julie thought the boys were cute, and they loved the black

Porsche. So when the boys asked them to pull over to talk, they agreed and turned into the next parking lot.

The boys introduced themselves as Mark and Todd and said they were from Dallas. The foursome talked for a few minutes, and then Todd suggested that Julie go with him in the Porsche and Mark with Stephanie in the Corvette. The girls agreed, and they made plans to meet back there in one hour. Stephanie drove off with Mark and they pulled into a Dairy Queen, at Mark's suggestion, for two 7-Ups. When they drove off, Mark asked if he could drive, and Stephanie reluctantly let him. He drove to a new subdivision and parked in the driveway of an unfinished house. They stepped out of the car and into the house, which had just been carpeted. Stephanie was apprehensive, but she later said that he was such an innocent-looking guy that she did not expect any trouble.

But trouble was what Mark had on his mind. He pulled a flask of bourbon from his hip pocket and a joint from his shirt pocket and offered both to Stephanie. Stephanie resisted and argued that her brother had trusted her with the car. She told him of the trouble she had been in and how she did not want to experience it again. But after some very successful plays, she drank her 7-Up with bourbon, accompanied by a few hits off the joint that Mark had lit up.

Once Stephanie tasted the bourbon, she wanted more. She guzzled it straight out of the flask. Then she smoked another joint with Mark. It was her first time ever to use marijuana. She felt very relaxed at first, but the combination of the Triavil, alcohol, and marijuana sent her out of control. Mark, sensing her condition, proceeded to unbutton her blouse and fondle her. She tried to fight him off, but she could not. He completely overpowered her and ripped all her clothes off. She was fighting furiously when he hit her repeatedly in the face, finally knocking her out. He raped her, then, just as she was coming to, he raped her again. Afterward he gathered up her clothes, put her in the car, and drove back to the parking lot where they had met. But on the way, Stephanie, who had passed out again, did not know he scraped the right side of the Corvette against a sign or a pole or another car, ripping off the chrome strips.

When Mark arrived at the parking lot, Julie and Todd were waiting. He screeched to a stop, leaped into the Porsche, and sped off with Todd. Julie ran to the Corvette and saw that Stephanie was nude and unconscious. She dressed Stephanie as best she could, then slapped her face repeatedly. She was relieved when Stephanie moaned and began to ask what had happened. Julie drove Stephanie back to her house, parked the car in the driveway, honked the horn, and ran off to find her way home. She did not want to be a part of what was about to happen.

It was just after eleven, and by this time Stansell was furious. When he heard the car's engine and the horn, he raced outside to find Stephanie in the passenger's seat. He also saw that the chrome had been ripped from the side of his car. He was furious. When he opéned the door to drag Stephanie out, he smelled the alcohol on her breath and the scent of pot on her clothes, which infuriated him even more. He dragged her on the lawn and started to slap her and shake her while he yelled, ''How could you do this?'' Every trace of the All-American boy had left him at that moment.

Thomas was awakened by the yelling and ran outside. He pulled Stansell off Stephanie as Stansell yelled for his father to look at the Corvette. But her father was looking at something else—his daughter. He could tell that she was drunk and that her clothes had been ripped. Cynthia joined them on the lawn. When she saw her beaten daughter, she began to cry. When Stansell realized how badly beaten her face was, he thought he had done it all and began to cry. Stephanie came to but could only mutter incoherently.

Stansell pulled the car into the garage and stayed with Stella while Cynthia and Thomas took Stephanie to the hospital. The emergency room doctor confirmed that Stephanie had been raped. He took some X-rays and did a complete examination to ensure that no further damage had been done. He recommended that Stephanie spend the night in the hospital. Cynthia stayed with her, and Thomas returned home to try to get some rest. His attempts were futile.

The next day Thomas brought Stephanie and Cynthia home. Thomas begged Stephanie to be absolutely honest with them so they could piece together the facts of what had actually happened. Honest was something that she had not been in previous discussions with her parents, but now there was no more reason to cover up. She told them what she remembered. She admitted to guzzling the bourbon and smoking the marijuana. She could remember her clothes being torn away. She was not sure, but she believed that she had been raped twice.

Thomas was stunned. He could not believe this was actually happening to him and his beautiful daughter. He was determined that it would never happen again. He felt certain that it would not have happened if Stephanie had not been drinking. He knew how strong she was and that she could have fought off almost anyone. The reality was painful, but he was not going to deny it any longer. He was going to take care of his daughter. He wanted her to get better, and he was willing to go to any length. Fortunately, Stephanie was at that point, also. Whatever it might take, she was willing to do it.

Thomas consulted the yellow pages and looked under *Alcohol & Drug Rehabilitation*. Our hospital was the first one he called. I was glad for that. Because that Saturday afternoon, Stephanie, still only sixteen years old, entered treatment for alcoholism, alongside fourteen men and two women, all at least twice her age. That treatment was the beginning of a new life for Stephanie and her family. Stephanie had grown up addicted. But now, at sixteen, she had a chance to grow up. And grow up she did.

CHAPTER THREE

STEPHANIE: REACTIONS AND ACTIONS

Growth occurred not only in Stephanie's life, but in the lives of all the Westmorelands. That growth process, so vital to continuing recovery from addiction, was fostered by the treatment team of that small Texas hospital: physicians, nurses, psychologists, therapists, and counselors. Each person was equipped with the knowledge about addiction that can dramatically change the progression of the problem.

Throughout the treatment process, requirements are placed on both the patients and their families. If these requirements are not met, treatment will not be successful. Probably the most important requirement, and one of the most difficult to meet, is complete honesty—honesty with self and with others. Until she entered treatment, Stephanie had been dishonest with everyone. Her mode of operation was to hide, deceive, cover up, and lie. Her family, in refusing to see the nature of her problem, had also been less than honest. Fortunately, the family was willing to change and face the reality of what had happened and what must happen for long-term recovery.

As the Westmorelands revealed more and more of what happened between the time Stephanie was ten and when she was almost seventeen, I was able to understand how the problem had crept up on Stephanie and infiltrated the family without anyone perceiving it. I also came to understand the problems and the reactions that allowed the addiction to progress. The reactions of the Westmorelands and those close to the problem were similar to how other families and significant others react to progressing addiction. Much can be learned in looking at these inappropriate, inconsistent, and at times, destructive reactions.

31

It is also valuable to examine alternatives that were available but not taken.

Reactions centering on the addiction process fall into three categories or types of problems. The first type of problem for the Westmorelands was a *thinking*, or informational, problem. This led to *feelings and emotions* that were harmful and did not lead to recovery. These thoughts and feelings formed the basis for *actions*, actions that enabled the problem to grow.

The Westmorelands were reacting to a problem that, according to a 1982 Gallup poll, affects more than one-third of all families. Yet in spite of epidemic proportions, there are thousands of people just like the Westmorelands who know absolutely nothing about the problem of alcoholism or drug addiction. This ignorance allows people to drink and use drugs and destroy lives almost without noticing. People take note at the point at which the evidence is so overwhelming that it can no longer be denied. But because of the lack of knowledge, needless destruction occurs within families, industry, and society.

Why does this ignorance about alcoholism and drug addiction continue in the midst of an epidemic that is mentioned in the headlines almost every day? How can a family live with an alcoholic 365 days out of the year and not suspect that alcohol is the source of the problem? The answer, pure and simple, is denial. Denial comes in several forms. One form is captured in the statement "It is not my problem." People do not seek out information because they refuse to assume responsibility to help correct the problem. Teachers say it is the parents' job. Parents say it is the schoolteachers' job. And as everyone stands around pointing fingers at each other, the problem continues to escalate.

For the Westmorelands, this was the case. They never discussed addiction, its signs and symptoms, because they assumed that the school system had handled it adequately. They knew nothing about the development, progression, and symptoms of addiction. They did not acquire the knowledge because they felt it was someone else's job to do that—and because of the second form of denial.

The second form of denial is best characterized by a statement made by Cynthia Westmoreland: "We thought that this happened to other people's children. We never dreamed that our daughter could have an addiction problem." This is a common attitude among parents—and among many industries and professions—preventing them from gaining the information needed to combat the problem. For instance, you might hear professional baseball or football team managers state that the problem "does not exist here." In other words: "Sure, some athletes have a problem, but not on my team." But in reality, no team or profession is exempt from the problem. Addiction treatment professionals pass around a letter that exemplifies this form of denial and why the ignorance flourishes. In this letter, a manager of a Los Angeles–area professional sports team makes the ultimate statement of denial. He says he does not believe there is any alcoholism in his particular sport. He believes this is so because of the physical demands placed on the players. He said they simply could not continue in the game with an alcohol problem. This was his rationale for not implementing a program to help the athletes who have developed an alcohol or drug problem. This manager is not alone in his beliefs. Many recent and widely publicized drug tragedies and scandals have brought about some change, but the denial still persists to a damaging extent.

Just as some in professional sports may think that athletes are exempt, other professions fall victim to the same beliefs. Airlines might state that it is a problem among physicians. Physicians might say that it is the corporate world which is being affected, not physicians. And corporate executives might state that although the boardroom is relatively free from the problem, the pilots are the ones who really need to do something about drugs and alcohol. And on it goes. As long as the denial and inaction continue, no one takes constructive steps to help those who have fallen victim to addiction.

If the belief is that it could never happen to "my" child or employees or profession, then denial will grow as the problem grows. If people do not believe it is a possibility, they will not ask the appropriate questions or seek the evidence that would either rule out or identify a chemical problem. The psychologist who thought Stephanie's problem was depression did not probe into the alcohol and drug areas enough to discover the alcohol problem. The minister never considered it important enough to discuss with either Stephanie or her parents. If both had thought of it as a possibility first, they might have acted to set up a system of recovery with Stephanie and the family. If they had realized how much denial is involved in an addiction problem, they might have spent the time and effort to discover the reality of Stephanie's alcohol usage. But if families and professionals do not sus-pect alcohol and drugs, they will not look for the evidence or ask the questions to uncover the true nature of the problem.

Probably the worst offender in Stephanie's case was the phy-sician. Instead of helping her and her family, he compounded the problem by trying to make things better on a short-term basis rather than considering what was needed in the long run. His prescription of Valium for Stephanie should never have been made without thoroughly going over Stephanie's alcohol and drug consumption. Since he failed to do that, he enabled the problem to progress to cross-addiction to alcohol and Valium. Though with the best of intentions, he introduced a young girl addicted to alcohol to a new addictive drug. The parents did not suspect that the Valium would be a problem, since it was pre-scribed by a physician.

Stephanie's parents also made another initial mistake. They clung to the initial belief that alcohol or drug problems happen to other people's children. Their naïveté could have been deadly for Stephanie. Even after Stephanie received the traffic citation for driving while intoxicated, they did not suspect alcoholism. And the police officers did not take the time to warn Thomas that his daughter probably had an alcohol problem. Thomas thought it was merely a one-time mistake; he could not imagine Stephanie in that situation again. Because he did not suspect alcoholism, he remained without information that could help Stephanie. He did not know one of the basic principles of deal-ing with alcohol and drug problems, which must be understood by parents, teachers, employers, and others close to the affected individual: *The problem is always worse than it appears to be*.

No matter where you are in the world or how extreme a per-son's drinking problem is, there is a standard answer to ''How much do you drink?'' Alcoholics everywhere usually reply, ''Just a couple of beers,'' or ''Just a few drinks.'' Whether your in-troduction to someone's problem drinking is such a statement or you discover empty bottles in the closet or beer cans under the car seat, it has to be assumed that only the tip of the iceberg is being seen. The problem needs to be assumed to be worse than what has been revealed on the surface. People concerned need to know this so that they can try to uncover data that ac-curately describe the drinking behavior. If that can be done, there is hope of knowing the extent of the problem and what to do to help resolve it.

The Westmorelands' informational problem was not unique. Knowledge about alcohol, drugs, and addiction is distorted by the myths and misconceptions spread at every level of society. When these misconceptions are confronted and changed, the likelihood of taking the most appropriate action increases greatly because the denial is destroyed. But society's attitudes, built on centuries of misinformation, are hard to change.

The stigma associated with alcoholism causes thousands of wasted lives because of the denial that it provokes. If people believe that alcoholics are skid row bums, no corrective action will be taken to help a beautiful, bright sixteen-year-old girl, or, say, a fifty-three-year-old top executive who has amassed millions of dollars. They couldn't be alcoholics! In fact, the popular skid row concept of the alcoholic applies to only 3 to 5 percent of them. The other 95 percent are left to progress toward that point because society is not aware that alcoholics can look like anyone and exist at any social level. The caricature in society's mind applies to a small percentage who have reached the late stages of the disease.

There are other destructive misconceptions and beliefs that have grown out of the alcoholic stigma. A common one is that the alcoholic is weak-willed and uses alcohol as a source of strength. In reality, alcoholics are some of the strongest-willed people in the world. Who else could drink a half bottle of vodka a day, work, and keep a family in the midst of growing stress with finances and legal battles? To be an alcoholic and continue to function requires a lot of strength. But no matter how strong the will or how well the alcoholic learns to cope, nothing will change the way the person drinks. No therapy has been designed to give that person a new body to metabolize the alcohol. The alcoholic's body will always be alcoholic. That is why quick fixes and magical cures neither solve the problem nor cure the alcoholic.

Other destructive beliefs about alcoholics are that they are immoral and that the drinking is a manifestation of an immoral life-style. Alcoholics undoubtedly do immoral things from time to time, but so do nonalcoholics. Even people who do not drink at all do immoral things. It is not surprising that an alcoholic who is addicted to a chemical, whose life is out of control, who obtains destructive information from an uninformed society will in desperation commit immoral acts. Once recovery begins, that immorality is removed and is replaced by acts of responsibility.

Many psychologists still hold the belief that the alcoholic is a victim of mental illness or that a personality disorder has produced the problem. That this is not true is strongly indicated by the large number of people who spend years in psychiatric treatment, are pronounced free of their mental illness, but still can't drink normally. It really is true that you may be able to change the alcoholic's thinking, but you will not change the alcoholic's drinking—it remains an all-or-nothing matter, with "nothing" the only survivable choice.

The most accurate and up-to-date information about alcoholics is that they are different from others. That difference is not a mental or spiritual one but a physical one. Alcoholics simply do not drink like most people. If society learns that, early identification will be easier, and help for the alcoholic will come sooner.

Help for Stephanie was delayed because of a standard misconception of parents about kids. The Westmorelands thought that "bad kids" had alcohol and drug problems; since Stephanie was not a bad kid, they did not look into the area of alcohol and drugs. If they had, their reactions to the progression could have helped her much sooner.

These issues are intensified by the confusion among professionals about what causes alcoholism and how to help someone who has it. One professional looks at the problem from one perspective, while another professional holds an entirely different view. This confusion is evident in how the professionals reacted to Stephanie's problem. The physician said it was adolescent adjustment difficulties, calling for allowing Stephanie time and more space. The teacher thought it was a lack of discipline, while the minister said it was a spiritual problem in need of an eternal solution. And the psychologist believed that at the root lay a depression in need of a mood-elevating chemical. Each one reacted differently, and each one allowed the problem to progress. Confusion among professionals can be deadly.

Confusion is rampant when the alcohol problem is broken down into three areas. Those areas are the use of alcohol, its misuse (problem drinking), and alcoholism.

On alcohol use, there are two extreme positions; both generate problems. One maintains that alcohol is a very poisonous chemical to all who consume it. People who hold this position believe that if a person drinks at all, destruction will eventually result. An example of this view is Cynthia Westmoreland's belief that all alcohol is evil and no good can ever come from it. If I had to pick an extreme, I would certainly pick this one. But observation does not bear out this view; in spite of the dangers of alcohol, it is evident that many people drink to some extent without experiencing or creating problems.

The extreme opposite of this view is that alcohol is a harmless substance to be enjoyed by everyone. Some even quote Scripture to the effect that it is the "gift of God that gladdens the hearts of men." To anyone who has worked with alcoholics, it is obvious that alcohol does not gladden everyone's heart—especially not the hearts of the family members. These extremes must be put aside if alcohol problems are to be resolved rather than reinforced.

Another informational problem is the difficulty people have distinguishing between alcohol misuse (problem drinking) and alcoholism. This difficulty causes many inappropriate reactions. I once heard a world-renowned alcoholism professional lecture on what an alcoholic is. He said that anyone who has a problem with alcohol in any way is an alcoholic. He said, for example, that if a fourteen-year-old girl drank one beer, rode her bicycle into traffic, and was hit by a truck, she was an alcoholic—because alcohol had affected her life in an adverse way. Thus, he went on to say, she was an example of an alcoholic who should never drink again.

Now, I am the first to say that if you want to know the reality of the problem, you must dig below the surface for accurate information. It *is* always worse than it appears. But if there are no other factors to this girl's problem, there is no evidence of alcoholism. She is a classic case of problem drinking. That she and the alcohol and the bicycle and the truck ended up in the same place at the same time is more an indication of bad luck than proof of alcoholism. As we will discuss later, alcoholism and problem drinking are in need of two totally different approaches. To build a strong foundation of recovery from alcoholism, society—and especially its professionals—must clarify its definitions and communicate accurately with those who need to know the facts about this problem.

It is only natural that many alcoholics, trapped in a deadly progression, do not know that they are alcoholic, and certainly do not know how to stop the progression. Alcoholism is, above all, insidious. Its early symptoms are almost invisible unless you know exactly what to look for. Alcoholics may think they are blessed with a high tolerance for alcohol, or later on they may believe they are becoming more and more neurotic, but it will take a lot of evidence and confrontation before they become willing to accept alcoholism as the problem. The denial will continue to destroy up to the last stages of the progression.

Alcoholic denial is fostered by criteria alcoholics establish for alcoholism. They are based on the acceptance of alcoholism as a stigma and on a lot of misinformation. Some common examples are:

"I'm not one if I can stop drinking any time."
"I'm not one if I don't drink every day."
"I'm not one if I don't drink during the day."
"I'm not one if I don't drink at work."
"I'm not one if I rarely get drunk."
"I'm not one if I can still control my drinking."
"I'm not one if I only drink beer."
"I'm not one if I only drink wine."
"I'm not one if I don't drink straight out of the bottle."
"I'm not one if my liver is in good shape."

These statements are based on misconceptions and prevent early detection and early action.

As the problem worsens, misconceptions become more deadly and delay the achievement of the desired outcome, sobriety. Inaccurate information and thoughts often damage alcoholics' ability to get well and recover. Familiar to almost every person with a drinking problem is the idea that "I can handle this alone." This is a natural response to everyone telling alcoholics that they must handle the problem, pull themselves together, show some willpower. Viewing alcoholism as a weakness results in the alcoholic trying to convince everyone of his or her personal strength, usually by exercises in controlled drinking. These futile attempts to demonstrate strength eventually fail. But until they do, the alcoholic will use anything available as evidence of being able to "handle my drinking." And while the alcoholic tries to manage the drinking, life becomes more and more difficult to manage.

The mismanagement of Stephanie's problem was caused by all these informational problems and beliefs. Misconception and indirection kept her from entering the recovery process before she was raped and beaten. Her own thoughts about alcohol and her problem were misguided. She viewed alcohol as both a source of fun and a sign of maturity. She thought she had discovered the secret of adulthood, but what she ultimately discovered was that her world was not equipped to help her with her problem. Her world had distorted reality and denied that more than just a "phase" was destroying her adolescent years and her future. She did not understand, and there was no one to help her understand. So she was left with a thinking problem. She possessed beliefs that allowed her to continue to drink for over six years before finally taking care of her problem. Ignorance and destructively inaccurate information all contributed to her thinking problem, just as every day it contributes to the thinking problem of society. If progress is to be made with the Stephanies among us, we must begin with new information, accurate information that sets the alcoholic free. Free, that is, to become anything except a "normal social drinker."

Misinformation contributed to Stephanie's problem reaching the crisis stage. No one knew how to resolve it; almost every reaction was destructive. Their thinking problem was not the Westmorelands' only handicap; it was compounded by emotions which eventually spun completely out of control. The entire family had to be treated before these inconsistent, destructive emotions could become manageable. They emerged as Stephanie's problem progressed to the middle and later stages. Before then, there were no feelings about alcoholism or drug addiction; they were nonexistent because of the denial of the severity of the problem.

The Westmorelands completely denied Stephanie's problem. The denial allowed them to avoid the emotional involvement required to resolve the problem. Human nature avoids pain at all costs, and the cost of accepting the painful reality of addiction is quite high. That is why so many for so long choose to avoid all emotional involvement with the addict and with the addiction.

Thomas served as a prime example of emotional disregard.

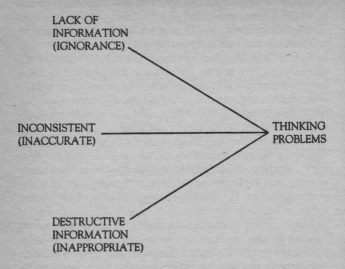

He expected Cynthia to handle Stephanie's problems at every stage of the progression. He remained detached and uninvolved with Stephanie and all the turmoil the family was experiencing. He knew nothing about alcoholism, and he did not want to know anything about it. As long as he chose the route of ignorance, he could remain a member of the family without paying the painful emotional price of facing reality. The reality was more painful, though: Thomas was losing his daughter and his family. As Stephanie and the family suffered with a problem they did not understand, Thomas drank beer and watched television.

Emotional disregard is a societal plague, preventing constructive, large-scale action to reduce the incidence of alcoholism and drug addiction. The vast majority do not know or care about the damage that results from alcohol and drugs. The Westmorelands' attorney represents this attitude of society. He did what he could to help reduce the discomfort of his clients, but by evading the consequences of Stephanie's drinking, the attorney allowed the Westmorelands to continue denying longer. The most helpful recommendation he could have made to the family would have been that Stephanie plead guilty and suffer the consequences of her actions. He did not do that because he was not willing to become emotionally involved with the family or with Stephanie's problem. His lack of knowledge allowed him to maintain his state of emotional disregard.

As Stephanie's problem progressed, so did the family's emotional intensity. Emotional detachment faded as the problem became more evident. Inconsistent and destructive feelings evolved from the incidents in Stephanie's life. Because of the drinking, Stephanie's behavior became a display of confusion and contradiction. Weeks of deviant behavior were interrupted by periods when Stephanie became the model child. This placed her family on an emotional roller coaster out of control. With the progression, it became more difficult to sort out whether what they felt for Stephanie was love, hate, guilt, fear, or anger. This inconsistency in feelings was another barrier to constructive action.

Alcoholic behavior never occurs in a vacuum. It always affects the people closest to the alcoholic. That is why the entire family, not just the alcoholic, must enter treatment. The treatment process can help the family deal with the inconsistencies in the ways they feel toward each other and the alcoholic. It was obvious how much Stephanie's family loved her, but hidden beneath the surface were feelings that erupted to overpower their love and concern. Stansell cared deeply for his sister, but as her behavior grew more extreme, he could not keep his anger in check. As he revealed in treatment, he developed a love-hate relationship with Stephanie. He had difficulty separating his love for her and his hatred for her behavior. To him, what she did was who she was. He hated what she did. That hatred of her behavior was evident on the night before she entered treatment, as he repeatedly slapped her out on the lawn. Once he saw her face and how badly she had been beaten, his anger turned to guilt. He felt brief guilt because he thought he had hurt her that badly, and more lasting guilt over not being able to change the course of events in her life.

Inconsistency was also evident in Stephanie's mother. She could not get a handle on her emotions. One moment she would feel like a loving wife and mother; the next, that she had become a destructive mother. She continually questioned where she had gone wrong. Believing that her mistakes had brought about Stephanie's problem, she experienced extreme guilt. The most painful emotion was her fear. She was afraid she was losing her daughter forever. She had no idea how to bring the situation under control. Every time she tried something, it produced a temporary change, but her hopes were constantly destroyed by each alcohol-related event. This emotional turmoil was more painful than anything Cynthia had ever experienced; at times she questioned her own sanity.

Every member of the Westmoreland family struggled with the extremes of emotions. The guilt and anger took a toll on the family and further complicated the problem, draining them of spontaneity and energy. The whole family became depressed under the weight of their predicament. This lack of energy and growing depression further negated the family's ability to act.

Stephanie experienced destructive feelings about herself. These feelings are common in most alcoholics who continue to drink. Initially, Stephanie was indifferent about her problem. She felt normal when she drank; it made her feel both mature and secure. She saw nothing negative in those feelings. But her drinking continued to cause problems for her. Even though she attempted to deny these problems, the evidence became too great. Her indifference turned into fear that she was not going to be "normal." She questioned her mental stability as she saw her life producing more and more problems for herself and those close to her.

Stephanie's feelings paralleled those of most alcoholics who are not recovering. She vacillated between the extremes of the emotional spectrum. These incompatible feelings that fought to override each other destroyed Stephanie's self-esteem. As her problem progressed, she would blame her parents for what she was experiencing; she would lash out at the way she was raised or point to her father's neglect. She would seize on anything that would absolve her of responsibility. But periods of blame and projecting her problem onto others were erased by times of overwhelming guilt. Her guilt feelings were deepest after she had hurt someone or failed to make progress in solving the problem herself. This guilt motivated her to seek relief from its pain; Stephanie always returned to the bottle for that relief. She knew that for a time it would shut out the world and shut off her emotions. To her it was the only means of escape, an alternative she could not refuse.

Stephanie's self-hatred and anger grew. She did not understand what was happening, and she was angry at not being able to control the problem. *For the alcoholic, where understanding does not exist, anger fills the void.* Stephanie's anger increased as each person interrupted her life to help but could not. As each attempt failed, she felt rejection and alienation from the world. She needed direction, but no one knew how to give it. The longer she struggled, the less hope she felt that she would ever be normal. Her emotions and her perceptions led her to believe that there was no way out; she was drowning in the booze and her own self-pity.

Stephanie's emotions were a predictable result of her drinking. The emotional distress of her family was also to be expected, given their ignorance of the problem and erroneous information about solving it. Their feelings could not be expected to be anything but destructive. The misinformation and the resulting emotions formed a troublesome foundation on which the Westmorelands' reactions were built. Inconsistent and destructive misinformation combined with inconsistent and destructive emotions could only result in inconsistent and destructive actions.

The third and final problem area for the Westmorelands was what they actually did: all the wrong things for the right reasons. They loved Stephanie, but misinformation and emotional turmoil led them to hurt her chances for recovery rather than help them. Their first reaction was to do nothing at all. They did not recognize the problem as alcoholism; they labeled it with other names and considered it in different ways. They did whatever was necessary to deny that Stephanie was an alcoholic. Stephanie was even more blind to the extent of the problem. She certainly could not correct a problem she did not believe she had; her family was in a much better position to intervene and take appropriate action.

Society often stands back and expects the alcoholic to make a radical change, motivated by some instantaneous insight. But this rarely happens. The alcoholic functions in a delusional world devoid of reality. Denial is strong, and rationalization accompanies each wrong step. Society condemns the drinking and the drinker without becoming involved in helping to solve the problem. Rarely will change occur until someone steps in to take control. The alcoholic really is powerless over the alcohol and

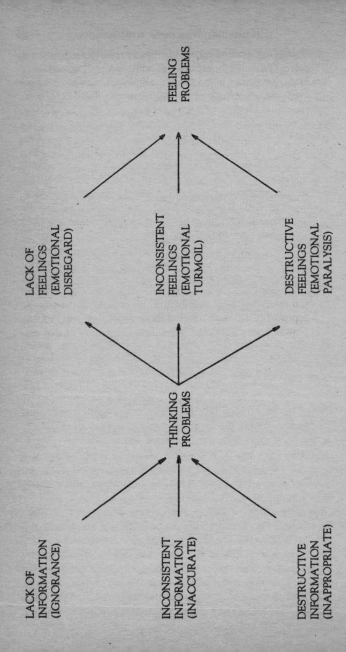

the driving force of addiction, and inaction and lack of intervention keep him or her in the grips of addiction and dependency.

Once others close to the alcoholic do take a risk and become involved, the actions are often inconsistent or destructive. One such action is to try to persuade the alcoholic to stop drinking. Stopping the drinking does not solve the problem. If someone is bleeding profusely from a deep gash in the arm, the appropriate advice is not to stop bleeding. The bleeding is evidence that help is needed. Stop the flow of blood and the wound is still subject to infection. It must be cleaned and mended. This parallels the needs of the alcoholic. Once the drinking is stopped, deep wounds remain within the alcoholic and the family; if these are not mended, it is only a matter of time before the alcoholic lapses back into drinking again.

Requesting that the alcoholic stop drinking only serves to aggravate the problem. Well-meaning people will guarantee that once the drinking stops, the other life problems will stop, but if the alcoholic does stop drinking, the chances are that life will be even more miserable than before. He or she will be without the dependable "friend" and without any other support. As withdrawal from the alcohol intensifies, the misery of that person will grow and will most likely be self-medicated with a return to the bottle. Once relief is felt, the alcoholic's belief that the alcohol is not the problem is strongly reinforced. What is needed goes beyond stopping drinking, there is a need for treatment that involves every member of the family.

This is why the psychologist's advice was very inappropriate in Stephanie's case. He could have seen the real problem if he had made the effort. He should have seen the need for the entire family to work together, but he never attempted to bring them into the therapy process. If Stephanie had made progress under his treatment, she would only have been thrown back into a sick family—a family that needed help just as much as she did.

When Cynthia tried to help, her actions arose from false hopes and unrealistic expectations. She hoped for a quick solution. She hoped that her minister could provide her daughter with a spiritual answer; then she sought out her physician's advice in hopes of a medical answer; finally, she reached out to a psychologist, hoping for a mental solution. Each of these attempts was flawed because they were one-dimensional. Of course Stephanie had a spiritual problem that needed to be dealt with;

but in addition, her emotional, physical, social, mental, and family difficulties needed to be handled. Hoped-for change would only come from a well-orchestrated plan of recovery that included every area of her life; a multidimensional solution was needed for a multidimensional problem. Acting on only one dimension left Cynthia frustrated and Stephanie's problem unaltered. She experienced temporary change but not long-term recovery.

Why didn't the Westmorelands act in a helpful way? *They were stuck*. They were stuck in thoughts, feelings, and actions that were sometimes inconsistent and often destructive. No one in the family could help Stephanie get unstuck because each of them was stuck in his or her own way. The family needed a different way of handling the problem, alternatives that would produce long-term results. But because of what they did not know and how they felt, their actions enabled the addiction to grow.

If Stephanie's drinking problem had occurred in a family and among professionals who knew about the problem and how to handle it, she would not have wasted her teen years suffering from a growing addiction. Thomas would not have waited so long before he acted to help his daughter. Cynthia would not have sought out professionals who could provide only one aspect of the solution. Neither Thomas or Cynthia would have been so vacillating in restricting Stephanie's activities and friends. They would have seen that inconsistency was only making matters worse. If Stansell had known, he would not have lied to his father about the extent of Stephanie's drinking. Stella would not have tried to cover up. The physician would not have prescribed a drug if he had been aware of the addiction process. The psychologist would not have treated Stephanie alone but involved the entire family. Those people did what they thought best to do, but because of their ignorance, what they thought best was not best; it was destructive and enabling (meaning that she was permitted to continue drinking).

What made the difference for Stephanie and the Westmorelands? They finally reached a point where they were willing to do anything. They entered treatment and learned a whole new way to think, feel, and act. They changed their thinking, resolved their emotional conflicts, and acted in a way that supported the long-term recovery of Stephanie and of themselves.

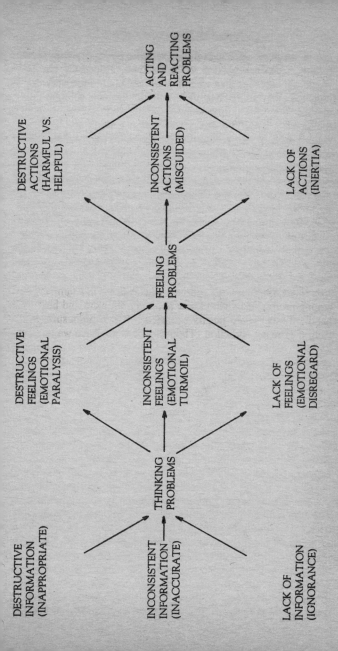

It was difficult, but it was better than the alternative of Stephanie continuing to drink until she could drink no more. Hope began with a change in the thinking process of every member of the family, but the effect did not end there. The Westmorelands influenced many families to take a look at what was happening with their children, to ask the difficult questions, and to develop the needed awareness to confront the alcohol and drug problem.

Growing Up Addicted is about people taking action to change society, one family at a time. This book contains the information needed for change. The insights negate some long-held beliefs and assumptions about addiction, but those beliefs, misperceptions, and myths have not helped us deal with this problem. Society as a whole has acted destructively because available information and attitudes toward the problem are destructive.

I hope that you are reading this book to learn and to change, to become a source of help, not harm. You and your family can realize the hope that was realized by the Westmorelands. And the Westmoreland story can be repeated in families across this country. Each of us must be willing to reach that point at which change can occur, that point where we are willing to do whatever it takes.

CHAPTER FOUR

THE CASE FOR PREDISPOSITION

A considerable amount of confusion has always surrounded alcoholism, its cause, and how it develops. Theories range all the way from demon possession to ordinal birth position. Unlike many other diseases and problems, no one has ever agreed on what causes alcoholism. As a result, the confusion has intensified over the years.

Central to the issue is the debate over "nature versus nurture." On one side are those who say that alcoholics are alcoholic from birth—or at least that at the time of birth, their "nature" or body is predisposed to developing alcoholism. Others argue that the alcoholic becomes so because of "nurture," or a problem in character or personality development. Accepting the "nature" view, one would say that there is a high rate of alcoholism in children of alcoholics because of an inherited susceptibility. The "nurture" stance would explain the high rate as learned behavior or the result of environmental influences. This theory strongly implies that alcoholism is caused by poor parenting. It also implies that alcoholism can be prevented through improved parenting. The argument over what causes alcoholism has gone on for years. All biases aside, where is the truth?

In my view, the evidence firmly supports the "nature" argument: alcoholism is very much a matter of inborn predisposition. The purpose of this chapter is to support this view by presenting both the results of scientific research and studies, and the observations I have made while working in treatment centers, churches, and counseling offices for the past ten years. In working with thousands of alcoholics and their families, I've had the good fortune to see most of those individuals and families recover. In this work, many conflicts have arisen over the cause and solution of alcoholism. What emerges as highly probable truth often is the opposite of the most widely held theories and beliefs. I hope that as you read on, you can wipe away any prejudice or bias and be objective as the information is presented. I have no ax to grind in championing this approach; it simply represents what I believe to be the truth about the problem of alcoholism.

One of the most common beliefs about alcoholism is that a certain alcoholic personality leads to the development of the problem—that some people have common personality traits that combine to produce an alcoholic. Another term that expresses the same belief is ''addictive personality.'' Both of these labels, alcoholic personality and addictive personality, indicate that a person's body becomes susceptible to alcoholism because of certain characteristics that originate in the mind. Although this is the most widely held belief, there is a big problem with it. When alcoholics come into treatment believing that their character, mind, or personality has produced the problem, there is a corollary hope that if the character, mind, or personality can be changed or improved, the alcohol problem will be resolved. That simply is not the case. Frequently a person in the early stages of recovery focuses on resolving personality conflicts, not in an effort to fully recover, but eventually to be able to resume normal social drinking. Of course, this always ends in relapse, and recovery is delayed. Thus it is an important element of treatment to confront an individual operating from the false assumption that if the personality produced the problem, there is hope for a cure by working on the personality. The alcoholic must be able to accept that no matter how spiritually strong or mentally healthy he or she becomes, it will not change his or her body. The body, if it drinks again, will drink as an alcoholic, regardless of the mental health of the individual.

In fact, there is no scientific evidence supporting the addictive personality concept. As published in *Alcoholism Report* (March 17, 1983), two studies conducted by the National Research Council of the National Academy of Sciences found absolutely no support for the existence of a personality profile that prefigures addiction.[1] This finding is supported in the treatment setting; patients' personalities simply do not manifest common traits that produce the problem. The confusion has arisen from observations made of those who are already into the addiction process. The early symptoms of alcoholism are invisible; it is not recognized until the person is well into the middle stage of addiction. When a person enters the addiction process and sets out to control that addiction, some very common and predictable *behaviors* and *reactions* will develop. These might include intense anger, low frustration tolerance, or compulsive behavior in other areas such as eating. These reactions and behaviors do not cause the problem, they are a result of the problem. *Thus what could be termed the "addicted" personality has been mistaken for a predisposing addictive personality that simply does not exist.*

Another closely related belief about alcoholism is that it is the result of a person attempting to cope with depression. The belief is that an extremely depressed individual will develop alcoholism as a result of poor coping mechanisms and the inability to deal with issues surrounding the depression. This idea is also a result of observing someone in the middle or latter stages of the addiction process rather than before the development of the process. It is understandable, since alcohol in large quantities is a central nervous system depressant; those who drink a lot of it will end up depressed. They will also be depressed over the tragedies that result from drinking over the years. Research shows that alcoholism produces severe depression as the problem progresses, but that depression is not a common condition for all alcoholics. It certainly is not a common preexisting condition that produces the problem.

Another commonly held belief is that environmental factors can lead a person into alcoholism. This theory holds that if an alcoholic had been brought up in a different situation, perhaps in a different home, the alcoholism could have been prevented. Much of the support for this belief comes from the fact that alcoholism does run in families. It is also reinforced by the undeniable fact that *drinking* is a learned behavior. Even *problem drinking* is a learned behavior. But *alcoholism* is inherited.

Cadoret, Cain, and Grove were involved in a study of adopted children raised apart from their biological parents. Their findings showed that *no environmental factors or socioeconomic standards of adoptive parents increased the risk for alcoholism in adoptees.*[2] This initial study pointed to the importance of the hereditary factor, not environmental, in the development of alcoholism. Many other studies support the same conclusion, that there is no one situation or environment that can be designated as a cause for alcoholism; even the role model of an alcoholic parent has nothing to do with the development of the problem. This finding was confirmed in studies of adoptees raised apart from their alcoholic biological parents. These children, born of alcoholic parents, were placed in homes, some of which proved to be alcoholic and some nonalcoholic. The study showed that whether the adoptee was placed with nonalcoholic or alcoholic adoptive parents made no difference in the incidence of alcoholism.[3] If alcoholism runs in families, but the presence of a practicing alcoholic parent does not enhance the probability of alcoholism, the logical area to examine as the source of the problem is genetics, heredity, and the concept of biological predisposition.

Some of the most prominent professionals in the field of alcoholism continue to negate the extensive amount of research pointing to a physiological basis for it. The reason for this is usually that there is no one conclusive study in the area of alcoholism and heredity—though many very convincing studies have been conducted. These studies, when examined together, point to the conclusion that alcoholism is caused from a physiological difference in the body of an alcoholic rather than some type of psychological difference in the mind. Each year, with added research, the evidence for predisposition mounts. Eventually, biological predisposition will no longer be denied as a factor in producing alcoholism.

In the Cadoret-Cain-Grove study, three indications from the adoptee research emphasize a biological susceptibility to alcoholism: (1) environmental factors explain less about the cause of alcoholism than do biological factors; (2) the addition of environmental factors to biological factors does not improve the predictability for alcoholism; (3) there is no evidence to indicate that environmental variables interact with biological variables to increase or decrease the risk for alcoholism in an adoptee with a biological familial background of alcoholism.[4] This is only one of several studies using adoption and placement records to study adoptees born to alcoholic and nonalcoholic parents. *These studies reveal alcoholism occurring with much greater than average frequency in those born to alcoholic parents, even when there was no contact with that parent after birth.*[5]

In 1978 Michael Bohman, M.D., completed a study of two thousand adoptees and their biological and adoptive parents. To conduct the study, he used the state criminal records and the official records of alcoholics. He also found a significant correlation between alcoholism in the biological parents and in their adopted-out sons. At the same time, his study failed to find any correlation between criminal parents and criminality in their biological children. So while failing to discover a correlation between parents and criminality, his study found one between alcoholic parents and alcoholic children. Again, the research supports a genetic explanation for the development of alcoholism.[6] This is especially significant since these children of alcoholic parents were raised apart from their biological mother and father. The genetic determinant for alcoholism was present.

Another study undertaken in 1978 by Cadoret and Gath reached the same conclusion. They looked at environmental variables that included socioeconomic status of the adoptive parents, psychiatric conditions in adoptive families, time spent in foster care before adoptive placement, and the age of the adoptee. The only significant predictor of alcoholism in the adoptee was a *biological* background of alcoholism.[7] Once again, strong evidence points away from personality and toward biological predisposition. It is irresponsible to deny the reality of these conclusions because of bias or prejudice toward alcoholics.

Two millennia ago, Aristotle declared that drunken women bring forth children like themselves; Plutarch said that one drunkard begets another; and nineteenth-century physician and researcher Benjamin Rush warned that parental alcoholism produced alcoholism in the offspring.[8] It appears that modern research supports the conclusions of these men. They may not have known the cause, but they observed the parental connection. The current evidence shows that this connection has a biological foundation. Not only does the parental alcoholism cause problems for the immediate offspring, but the susceptibility that they inherit is passed from generation to generation, even if there is an intervening generation or so of teetotalers. It is not the drinking *behavior* that is inherited, so even if members of one generation do not drink, the biological predisposition can be handed down to the next. A study by Lennart in 1975 indicated that there was a threefold additional risk of alcoholism through the fifth decade of life for grandchildren of alcoholics.[9]

One of the best-known researchers in the area of alcoholism and genetics is Donald Goodwin, M.D., who has probably done more than anyone else to call attention to the influence of genetics on alcoholism. In 1973 Goodwin and his associates completed a study of adoptees raised apart from their biological parents. *The sons of alcoholic biological parents had a much greater incidence of alcohol problems than those of nonalcoholic parents.* The groups did not differ in any other way; there was no greater incidence of depression or character disorders. The only difference was the increased rate of alcoholism among sons of alcoholics.[10]

In 1974, Goodwin's study of drinking problems in adopted and nonadopted sons of alcoholics was reported. In this study, the sons of alcoholic parents who were adopted in infancy were compared with brothers raised by an alcoholic parent. The findings revealed that the length of exposure to the alcoholic parent had nothing to do with the development of alcoholism. It was also discovered that the severity of the parent's alcoholism, determined by the number of hospitalizations, was positively related to alcoholism in the offspring. The main finding was that sons of alcoholics are no more likely to be alcoholic if raised by their biological parents than if they were taken out of the home during infancy.[11] It is difficult to review the work done by Goodwin and not grasp the significant evidence for a genetic cause for alcoholism. In addition, it points to the fact that, *other than the genes that parents pass on, they do not contribute to alcoholism in their children.* A parent who feels guilty over an alcoholic son or daughter has no reason to blame himself or herself.

A recent study reported in the August 30, 1982, bulletin of the NIAAA Information and Feature Service supports Goodwin's adoption studies. The study was made in Sweden, using the medical records of 862 adopted males and 913 adopted females. The conclusions of the study were that if the biological parent was alcoholic, the children ran a greater risk than average of also being alcoholic; if the natural parents were not alcoholic and the adoptive parents were, the risk was not increased. This study not only supports other research reported but also indicates that parents living with a tremendous weight of guilt, feeling that they have caused their children to be alcoholic by the way they raised them, have no basis for their self-blame.[12] This is yet another example of research conducted with adoptees that supports the strong hereditary influence in the development of alcoholism. Research in other areas is now supporting the same conclusions about biological predisposition.

Scientists studying brain waves believe that sons of alcoholic parents may be genetically susceptible to alcoholism. Their research presents the first purely biological evidence for alcoholism being hereditary. Under the direction of Dr. Floyd Bloom of the Alcohol Research Center at the Salk Institute in La Jolla, the researchers found that the brain waves of sons of alcoholic parents were different from those of sons of nonalcoholic parents. Using brain wave comparisons, they were able to determine with 80 percent accuracy which sons were from alcoholic homes or nonalcoholic homes. They noted that the brain wave differences had a biological basis and were not the result of the alcoholism. The study suggests a genetically determined predisposition to alcoholism on a pharmacodynamic basis.[13] This certainly substantiates the case for genetic alcoholism, but it also may serve as a predictor of alcoholism and thus be used as a strong prevention tool.

The brain wave study is just one of many research efforts directed at finding an indicator for high susceptibility to alcoholism. The search for a genetic marker has increased in the past few years. In the past, studies with this objective have been widely varied. Color blindness, blood groups, proteins, and even finger ridge counts have been investigated.[14] But now studies are focused on the genes of alcoholic families. The hope is that one day a chromosome test can reveal a high level of susceptibility to alcoholism, which would serve as an effective preventive tool.

In seeking answers to the question of why some become alcoholic and some do not, it becomes obvious that certain individuals react differently to alcohol than do others. Wolf, in his study on ethnic differences in alcohol sensitivity, presented some statistics that indicate a person's susceptibility to alcoholism may be based on ancestry. In comparing the reactions to alcohol of Mongoloid (Japanese, Taiwanese, Korean) and Caucasoid adults, the results differed noticeably. Eighty-three percent of the Mongoloid adults responded to drinking alcohol with a marked visible flush. Only one of 34 Caucasoid adults flushed visibly. The study was expanded to include infants to ensure that drinking history did not influence the findings. When alcohol was administered to the Mongoloid infants, 74 percent had a visible flush. Only one of 20 Caucasoid infants had a visible flush. The report states that the response to drinking and symptoms of intoxication may prevent certain ethnic groups from consuming even moderate amounts of alcohol.[15] This inherited reaction to the chemical may prevent some groups from experiencing a high rate of alcoholism and enhance the rate in other groups. If the initial reaction to small quantities of alcohol is unpleasant, the likelihood of a drinking problem developing is much less. One important aspect of the study is that it underscores the fact that everyone does not react to alcohol in exactly the same way. You cannot generalize when talking about alcohol's effect on the body. It varies greatly from person to person.

Information closely related to this study was reported by the *World Press Review* in August of 1981: scientists had recently discovered that an enzyme found in the Japanese was responsible for their reaction to alcohol. The population has a low rate of alcoholism, for which the researchers concluded that the Japanese people's own body chemistry was responsible. Studies at the Center for Alcohol Studies at the University of North Carolina revealed that the DBH enzyme appears at differing levels in different people, and those levels correlate closely to the varying responses to alcohol. This study indicated that the more of the enzyme present, the better the feeling from the drinking and the greater the capacity to consume alcohol.[16] All these reports lead to the conclusion that there is more to the drinking phenomenon and the development of alcoholism than what occurs in the mind of the drinker. Alcoholism cannot be understood without the knowledge that reaction to alcohol differs greatly among individuals because of biological factors beyond the control of the drinker. The alcoholic begins drinking for the same reasons that others drink, but because of a faulty ''drinking machine'' or system, the alcohol reacts with the body in a different way to produce drastically different results.

A system develops a susceptibility to alcoholism in ways other than strictly through the genetic process. In cases of mothers who drink heavily during pregnancy, there have been births where infants have gone into withdrawal as soon as the umbilical cord was cut, because of the alcohol content of the mother's blood, which up to that moment had been nourishing the fetus. It really is true that when the mother gets drunk, the unborn baby does also. By the time of birth, the newborn is addicted. When this individual takes a drink years later, the addiction will be reactivated, and that drink will produce a different reaction than if the child had been carried by an abstinent mother. *Studies of mammals have indicated that offspring exposed to alcohol either* in utero *or during lactation have stronger alcohol preferences later.*[17] This preference factor is probably due to the addiction process started while the mammal was still in the womb. This is yet another important item of information for those who believe that alcoholism is a self-inflicted problem. There are simply too many factors that indicate that it is not so.

Since evidence points toward a genetic basis for alcoholism, it is important to look at the chemical makeup of the alcoholic to discover any observable differences. If alcoholism is inherited, there should be some observable chemical indications that verify the supposition that the alcoholic's system metabolizes the alcohol differently than the normal drinker's. One of the most fascinating chemicals that has been discovered as a link to alcoholism is tetrahydroisoquinoline, or THIQ. There are certain strains of laboratory mice that have been bred to have a thorough dislike for alcohol. In fact, these mice would rather die of thirst than drink a solution of water and vodka. But when the mice were injected with just a small amount of THIQ, their distaste for alcohol turned into a preference for it. The more often the THIQ was injected, the more the craving for alcohol intensified. This craving persisted for months afterward. This indicates that a minor chemical change in the brain of an alcoholic could lead to increased craving of alcohol and that the craving would persist long after the drinking has stopped.[18] How does this chemical enter and accumulate in the brain of the alcoholic?

In Houston, Texas, medical researcher Virginia Davis was doing cancer research using the brains of individuals who had recently died, many of them "winos" who had died the night before. When she began testing the brains of the alcoholics who had died on the streets, she discovered a heroinlike substance and concluded that the winos, in addition to their addiction to alcohol, were addicted to heroin. Well, if you know much about the 5 percent of alcoholics classified as winos, you know that they barely have enough money to purchase the cheapest bottle of wine, much less being able to support an expensive heroin habit. As Virginia Davis continued her study, she discovered that this highly addictive chemical she had found was THIQ. Further study indicated that in the body of the alcoholic, something occurs that does not happen in a normal drinker.

In a normal drinker, alcohol is converted into the very toxic chemical acetaldehyde. A large enough buildup of this substance causes death, so the body quickly turns it into acetic acid. After a series of other changes, the drinker is left with carbon dioxide and water, which are eliminated through the kidneys and the lungs. Within the system of the alcoholic, something else occurs. Not all the acetaldehyde is eliminated. The small amount that stays in the body winds up in the brain. There it undergoes chemical changes and ends up as the substance called THIQ.

This chemical is probably one of the main culprits in the development of alcoholism. For one thing, it does not occur in the brain of the nonalcoholic drinker; for another it is highly addictive in nature. During World War II, it was tried as a painkiller but had to be abandoned because it was proven to be more addicting than morphine. Third, once this chemical is in the brain, it stays there. A study of monkeys injected with THIQ revealed that the chemical was still in the brain seven years later.[19]

So a person who was biologically predisposed to alcoholism could begin drinking innocently just like anyone else, but as he or she continues to drink, the THIQ chemical begins to build up in the brain, causing the addiction process to intensify. Eventually the person becomes hooked on alcohol just as a heroin user would be hooked on heroin. Once the addiction is there, the alcoholic is on a progression toward total loss of control, and that loss of control can lead to other addictions as the alcoholic attempts to treat the alcohol addiction with sedatives and other addictive chemicals. Again, it is important to note that *the alcoholic begins drinking for the same reasons as anyone else, but ends up trapped by the addiction process because of biochemical changes unique to the alcoholic.*

Further support for the biochemical basis for alcoholism comes from a study of children of alcoholics. Compared to a control group with nonalcoholic parentage, the children of alcoholics had elevated levels of acetaldehyde after consuming a single dose of alcohol. The fact that there was a marked difference in the metabolism is significant enough, but the report went on to state that this higher level of acetaldehyde may facilitate the formation of condensation products with monoamine metabolites. These substances would promote the production of the addicting morphinelike alkaloids.[20] Thus a predisposed individual who takes one drink of alcohol does not get one drink's worth of addictive chemical but a stronger addictive dose because of the metabolic differences.

Donald Goodwin, genetic researcher, relates the following in his book, *Is Alcoholism Hereditary?*: "By 1980, at least a dozen groups of investigators were studying the children of alcoholics-non-adopted as well as adopted and comparing them with children of nonalcoholics. These were the findings:

1. Children of alcoholics have a higher tolerance for alcohol than do children of nonalcoholics.
2. Children of alcoholics underrespond to certain stimuli recorded on electroencephalograms (EEGs)
3. Children of alcoholics generate more alpha activity on the EEG.
4. Children of alcoholics are more often hyperactive than other children."

The key elements of the findings are that tolerance is greater for those with a genetic link to alcoholism.*

The correlation between high alcoholism rates in children of alcoholics and the finding of a difference in the processing of the alcohol within the system of those children underscores both genetic predisposition and the biological susceptibility factors leading to alcoholism. In making the case for biological predisposition and susceptibility, we must address the concept of tolerance in relation to the development of alcoholism. On the subject of tolerance, society has been a very poor teacher. If you ask people at random to define what an alcoholic is, many will tell you that it is someone with a low tolerance for alcohol. Encountering a woman drunk on one glass of wine and a man who has consumed two pitchers of beer without showing any signs of intoxication, most would identify the woman as being

*Donald W. Goodwin, M.D., *Is Alcoholism Hereditary?* (New York: Ballantine, 1988) 4.

highly susceptible to alcoholism; many would say that a man who can hold his alcohol is not an alcoholic and that the single most important factor in determining whether or not someone is alcoholic is the ability to control the drinking. These false assumptions have prolonged the suffering of many people.

In working with thousands of alcoholics, I've seen only one characteristic that they all had in common: the ability to consume vast quantities of alcohol. It was only in the latter stages of the progression that the tolerance began to drop off significantly. Lemere, back in 1956, reported in the *American Journal of Psychiatry* that in spite of repeated attempts to identify and delineate the alcoholic personality, only one trait is common to all alcoholics, *and that is the ability to drink too much.*[21] Although it is rather a simple observation, it is an insight that has escaped many.

Research by Cloninger and his associates reveals that predisposition is largely a genetic phenomenon, and before alcoholism is evident, continued heavy drinking is required.[22] In addition, research at the Finnish Foundation for Alcohol Studies also determines that the frequency and quantity of alcohol consumption have a substantial heritability.[23] Thomas Lipscomb and Peter Nathan, in researching blood alcohol level discrimination, present the possibility of an inherited predisposition for the acquisition of tolerance.[24]

These findings are significant in light of the mistaken assumption that tolerance is acquired mainly from the practice of heavy drinking. The common belief is that the more you drink, the more you will need to drink. With other chemicals such as opiates, this is true, but not with alcohol. In clinical studies, animals given repeated doses of alcohol fail to show any acquisition of a higher tolerance level. When young men with no prior drinking experience were administered doses of alcohol, their response to the drink varied widely. Some felt no effect, while others became quite intoxicated. This study demonstrates that tolerance does not correlate with prior drinking experience. The only explanation that accounts for the differing tolerance levels and the ability to acquire tolerance is that innate biological factors are responsible.[25]

In 1981 at the International Conference on Alcoholism and Drug Dependence in Liverpool, England, the results of a project were presented that supported the genetic determination of tolerance. The study found that the level of alcohol intake in both males and females is strongly influenced by inherited factors.[26] A study of 902 pairs of Finnish male twins reached the same conclusion. The identical twins, possessing the same genetic code as their brothers, were concordant in both quantity and frequency of drinking. The researchers found a heritable influence for the ability to consume alcohol.[27] A similar study by Jonsson and Nilsson, using 7,500 pairs from Sweden, found that identical twins were highly harmonious with regard to the quantity consumed. Evidence clearly shows that a person cannot merely choose to drink a lot of alcohol. There are factors far beyond choice that control the level of intake of alcohol for each individual.

Tolerance does not refer only to the amount that a person can consume. It also refers to the behavioral effect that the alcohol has on the drinker. A person with a high tolerance for alcohol will not only be able to drink a lot, but it will also take a lot of alcohol to produce the same effect that other drinkers experience with very little alcohol. This decreased reaction to the alcohol has also been shown to have a direct correlation to family histories of alcoholism.

Marc A. Schuckit, director of research of the Alcohol Treatment Program at the Veterans Administration Medical Center in San Diego, studied the reactions of men with and without family histories of alcoholism. He found that the two groups reacted quite differently when given three or four drinks of alcohol. The men from alcoholic families were much less physically and mentally impaired. In men with no family history of alcoholism, the level of impairment from the drinks was much greater.[28] What is inherited appears to be the ability to drink a lot of alcohol and feel less from it than a normal drinker would. The person susceptible to alcoholism is the one who appears to be "blessed" with the ability to drink. The fellow who can drink everyone under the table is the same one who will eventually experience the consequences of alcoholism. The insidious feature is that those consequences will not present themselves until later in the progression of the problem. By that time there will be a tremendous amount of evidence that the alcoholic can control the drinking. The only hope will come when that person realizes that the ability to control drinking is *not* a sign of a normal drinker. More and more it appears that society's view of alcoholism is in direct conflict with the actual facts.

Normal drinkers cannot drink the amount of alcohol necessary for alcohol to become a major problem. A normal drinker can have all sorts of other problems, but the drinker must be able to drink a great deal of alcohol in order for alcohol to be the central problem. What normal drinkers have that the alcoholic does not have is called an automatic limiting mechanism. If a person becomes very sick or uncontrollably drunk on one glass of wine, the ability to drink a lot has obviously not been inherited.

Goodwin states that it is essential to be able to drink large quantities of alcohol to be alcoholic. He has discovered that innate cutoff points, or automatic limiting mechanisms, prevent many from drinking large amounts. The innate cutoff points are determined by alcohol metabolism rates. And identical-twin studies show that metabolism rates are genetically determined.[29] It appears that both the ability and inability to drink are genetic.

In a study of drinking patterns of women, Goodwin determined that many women are physiologically susceptible to the adverse effects of drinking. The moderate drinking he found in the women was accompanied by headache and nausea when attempts were made to consume larger quantities. Of the women he studied who drank immoderately, most developed problems with their drinking that eventually required treatment.[30] Bohman and his associates also conclude that many women are more likely to avoid heavy consumption because of the adverse effects of the alcohol.[31] So why are there more men than women in treatment for alcoholism? Is it due to environmental stresses or the traditional male role model? Perhaps it is due to the greater susceptibility to alcoholism of men than women.

The conclusions of Goodwin's 1979 study form a basis for understanding alcoholism as a genetic phenomenon. In that study Goodwin states that to be alcoholic, you must be able to drink a lot of alcohol. He also states that there is a genetic predetermination whether a person will experience mild, intense, or no euphoria from drinking. In addition to the euphoria that the alcoholic experiences, there is a dysphoric effect—anxiety, dissatisfaction, restlessness—which is more readily found in the alcoholic than in the normal drinker. This dysphoric effect reinforces the person's continued drinking to override the discomfort.[32] So the alcoholic, expecting to drink normally and experience the same effects as normal drinkers, finds that something different occurs. The alcoholic can drink more, and when the drinking subsides, the adverse effects are much greater. These adverse effects reinforce continued drinking. The alcoholic finds himself or herself in the grips of the addiction process with little realization that something is drastically wrong. By that time, the drinking will have produced such a delusional world for the alcoholic that he or she will be genuinely trapped by the drinking.

The reason for this lengthy presentation on the genetic predisposition for alcoholism is partly that few people are aware of the vast amount of evidence supporting a biological susceptibility to alcoholism. More important, as a foundation of understanding the problem, this knowledge can assist the alcoholic in recovery. So many alcoholics don't begin recovery because of guilt and shame and remorse over the past. The family and society have reinforced the belief that the alcoholism is self-inflicted and that the alcoholic should be able to stop the drinking and produce a normal life immediately. When alcoholics are able to see the problem from the proper perspective, they are able to handle the guilt in manageable doses. This is so important because a person begins recovery not when he or she feels guilt over the past, but when he or she accepts responsibility for today—not for having caused the problem, but responsibility for getting over that problem. The only way to get over the problem is to put the past in perspective and begin the process of totally recovering the life to which the alcoholic is entitled, and that is a life free of addiction and full of purpose.

It is time for those who really want to do something about alcoholism to put aside their old beliefs about the problem and look at the facts. Research stacked upon research points to a genetic factor that is a predeterminant of alcoholism. For too long people have looked at the personality of the alcoholic after alcoholism has been present for years and said that the personality is the cause. But looking at the result of the addiction does not point to its root. Additional confusion is created because of the distinct difference in the nature of alcoholism and the behavioral problem known as problem drinking. Problem drinking can be learned; it is a choice. But alcoholism is something much deeper. It is found in the very nature of a person's physiology.

The value of this concept is twofold. If an alcoholic can be identified even before the first drink is consumed, there are all sorts of possibilities for prevention. Prevention can also be facilitated if people recognize heavy drinking for what it is. It is not an indication of mental or psychological strength but a symptom of alcoholism. It is the ability to drink a lot with little effect that forms the foundation of alcoholism. The other value to this concept is in the treatment of the problem. Too many people never recover because of their enormous guilt over being alcoholic. This concept frees them to accept responsibility to get well rather than try to become good. The goal is not guilt over the past but action toward the future.

The research and personal experience with alcoholism reveal what does *not* cause alcoholism. It is not caused by a set of personality traits called an addictive personality. The personalities of alcoholics vary greatly before they start drinking. Because of addiction, there are similar reactions during the progression of alcoholism. But once the alcoholic begins recovery, the personality varies greatly from those of other alcoholics. The similarities lessen as the real person emerges from the addiction.

Alcoholism is not caused by depression, either. Alcohol is a depressing chemical to the central nervous system and produces many depressed drinkers. But alcoholism is not a reaction to depression; depression is merely a common symptom of it.

Alcoholism is not caused by a spiritual weakness. People who are not spiritually strong are not predisposed to alcoholism. They may feel empty and purposeless and as a result drink, but that does not cause alcoholism. Alcoholism instead causes spiritual weakness. It tears a person from God and any ability to grow spiritually or increase in knowledge of God.

Environment does not cause alcoholism. An environment may lead to problem drinking and the need to escape, but no environment causes alcoholism. Rich and poor, good parents and ineffective parents all have alcoholism among their children. There will never be an environment that allows immunity from alcoholism. Neither parents nor the home can be marked as the source of alcoholism's development. Socioeconomic status, income levels, neighborhoods, states, and countries are all irrelevant to who becomes alcoholic and who does not. No psychiatric problem or psychological dilemma produces an alcoholic.

Alcoholism is caused by a combination of factors that produce a liability to the disease. *These are all physiological in nature;* they occur in the body, not in the mind. The body of the alcoholic does not have an automatic limiting mechanism. Whereas a normal drinker becomes sick or drunk from a lot of alcohol, the alcoholic is able to continue to drink. The alcoholic body develops a tolerance for alcohol that the nonalcoholic does not have.

The ability to drink a lot compounds the addiction problem with a faulty metabolism, which can produce a chemical, THIQ, that can be more addictive than heroin. The difference in metabolism can come from ethnic or racial differences, but, whatever the source, the alcoholic has a different system from that of the nonalcoholic. He has an innate ability to drink a lot and feel less effect than the nonalcoholic. He or she is the victim of a syndrome that few people understand.

Considerable evidence points to the fact that alcoholism is genetically influenced. Animal studies show that animals can be bred to have a greater or lesser sensitivity to alcohol. Family studies show that sons and daughters of alcoholics are at far greater risk than others for developing alcoholism. Twin studies show that the identical twin of an alcoholic has a 60 percent greater risk for alcoholism. A fraternal twin, with less genetic similarities, is only at 30 percent greater risk. Adoption studies show that no matter what the environment, sons and daughters of alcoholics are more susceptible to alcoholism. All these studies show a genetic influence, an inherited susceptibility to the problem.

One final point needs to be added to balance the biological susceptibility concepts presented here. It really does not matter what new research is conducted to document the cause of alcoholism. It may help in prevention, and with some guilt in recovery. But recovery from alcoholism is the same, no matter what caused the problem. It will always involve the same actions and the same principles. The guilt may, mercifully, be less, but recovery will be the same. It will always involve a daily decision to stop drinking, one day at a time.

NOTES

1. *The Alcoholism Report*, vol. XI, no. 10 (17 March, 1983): 6.
2. Remi J. Cadoret, M.D., Colleen A. Cain, and William M. Grove, "Development of Alcoholism in Adoptees Raised Apart from Biological Relatives," *Archives of General Psychiatry* 37 (May 1980): 561–76.
3. Donald W. Goodwin, M.D. et al., "Alcohol Problems in Adoptees Raised Apart from Alcoholic Biological Parents," *Archives of General Psychiatry* 28 (February 1973): 243.
4. Cadoret, Cain, and Grove, "Alcoholism in Adoptees," 563.
5. Center for Alcohol Studies, Chapel Hill, North Carolina, *Genetic Factors in Alcoholism*, vol. 1, no. 1, September 1980.
6. Michael Bohman, M.D., "Some Genetic Aspects of Alcoholism and Criminality," *Archives of General Psychiatry* 35 (March 1978): 268.
7. Remi J. Cadoret, M.D., and Ann Gath, "Inheritance of Alcoholism in Adoptees," *British Journal of Psychiatry* 132 (1978): 252–58.
8. Donald W. Goodwin, M.D., "Alcoholism and Heredity," *Archives of General Psychiatry* 36 (January 1979): 57–61.
9. Lennart Kaij and Jan M. Dock, "Grandsons of Alcoholics," *Archives of General Psychiatry* 32 (November 1975): 138.
10. Goodwin, et al., "Alcohol Problems in Adoptees," 243.
11. Goodwin, et al., "Alcohol Problems in Adoptees," 243.
12. Nancy Johnson, *NIAAA Information and Feature Service*, 30 August, 1982.
13. P. Propping, J. Kruger and N. Mark, "Genetic Disposition to Alcoholism. An EEG Study in Alcoholics and Their Relatives," *Human Genetics* 59 (1981): 51–59.
14. Donald W. Goodwin, M.D., "Genetic Components of Alcoholism," *Annual Review of Medicine* 32 (1981): 94.
15. Peter H. Wolf, "Ethnic Differences in Alcohol Sensitivity," *Science*, 28 January 1972, 450.
16. Center for Alcohol Studies, *Genetic Factors in Alcoholism*, 2.
17. H. L. Rosett, "Clinical Pharmacology of the Fetal Alcohol Syndrome," in vol. 2 of *Biochemistry and Pharmacology of Ethanol*, ed. E. Majchrowiez and E. P. Noble (New York: Plenum Press, 1979), 485–509.
18. Center for Alcohol Studies, *Genetic Factors in Alcoholism*.
19. David L. Ohlms, M.D., *The Disease Concept of Alcoholism* (Belleville, Ill.: Gary Whiteaker, 1983) 17.
20. "Ethanol Ingestion: Differences in Blood Acetaldehyde Concentrations in Relatives of Alcoholics and Controls," *Science*, 5 January 1979, 54.
21. F. Lemere, "The Nature and Significance of Brain Damage from Alcoholism," *American Journal of Psychiatry* 113 (1956): 361–62.

22. Robert Cloninger, M.D. et al., "Implications of Sex Differences in the Prevalences of Antisocial Personality, Alcoholism and Criminality for Familial Transmission," *Archives of General Psychiatry* 35 (August 1978): 948.

23. J. Partanen, K. Brunn, and T. Markanen, *Inheritance of Drinking Behavior. A Study of Intelligence, Personality, and Use of Alcohol of Adult Twins*, Alcohol Research in Northern Countries, ser. 14 (Helsinki: Finnish Foundation for Alcohol Studies, 1966).

24. Thomas R. Lipscomb and Peter E. Nathan, "Blood Alcohol Level Discrimination. The Effects of Family History of Alcoholism, Drinking Pattern & Tolerance," *Archives of General Psychiatry* 37 (May 1980): 576.

25. Goodwin, "Alcoholism and Heredity," 60.

26. J. B. Saunders, "Alcoholism: New Evidence for a Genetic Contribution," *British Medical Journal* vol. 284, no. 6323, 1137–38.

27. Partanen, Brunn, and Markanen, *Inheritance of Drinking Behavior*, 93.

28. "Groups Found to Differ in Reaction to Alcohol," *NIAA Information and Feature Service*, 31 December 1981.

29. Goodwin, "Alcoholism and Heredity."

30. Donald W. Goodwin, M.D., et al., "Psychopathology in Adopted and Non-adopted Daughters of Alcoholics," *Archives of General Psychiatry* 34 (September 1977): 1008.

31. Michael Bohman, M.D., Soren Sigvardsson, and C. Robert Cloninger, M.D., "Maternal Inheritance of Alcohol Abuse—Cross Fostering Analysis of Adopted Women," *Archives of General Psychiatry* 38 (September 1981): 969.

32. Goodwin, "Alcoholism and Heredity."

CHAPTER FIVE

DISPELLING THE MYTHS OF ALCOHOLISM

What people think about alcohol, alcoholics, and alcoholism is filled with myths and untruth. This major addiction problem continues to ravage families because of the stigma attached to the problem. The stigma supports the need for denial and covering up the problem. It also allows a person to be caught in the middle of the addiction process and not be aware that the increasing problems are a result of drinking. In many circles, alcoholism has remained a moral issue. Certain groups view the alcoholic's life as a result of immorality. Still others would classify it as a manifestation of underlying unresolved psychosocial issues. The opinions vary from profession to profession.

Everyone has been affected by the myths of alcoholism. Each person holds on to some cherished belief about the cause of alcoholism or how to cure it. It is very difficult to give up long-held thoughts and emotions about this problem. It is much more comfortable to stick with what has been believed for generations. But this is a new era. The time is right to take a fresh look at alcoholism and the people who suffer from it. The myths must be discarded and replaced with reality that comes from current research and the experience of thousands of alcoholics who have recovered from it.

This chapter is intended to shed new light on an old problem. It presents some widely held—but false—beliefs about alcoholism. After each myth is a brief summary of what I believe to be the most accurate and current information available. It may be difficult to accept this information because it counters so many popular misconceptions. In any case, it should be considered as only a beginning point for reconsidering this deadly problem;

what is introduced here will be further explained and supported in the subsequent chapters or has been in previous ones.

There are thirty major myths, which fall into four categories:

Alcohol and drinking
Alcoholics and drinkers
Alcoholism
Stopping drinking and recovery

MYTHS ABOUT ALCOHOL AND DRINKING

1. Alcohol is a depressant to the central nervous system. Like other depressant chemicals, its initial effect is to depress the activity of the central nervous system. Therefore, alcohol would be classified as a "downer" drug.

If you observe a party where alcohol is being served, during the first hour you are not likely to see the appearance of mass depression. Depression is not characterized by loud talking, laughter, and people having fun. If the chemical's initial effect was depressing, you would see depressed behavior. But instead of depression, the evidence indicates stimulated activity. How can a depressant of the central nervous system produce a stimulating effect?

The answer is simple. Alcohol has initial stimulating effects that later give way to the depressing properties of the chemical. Unlike other drugs, such as Valium or Librium, alcohol contains calories. These calories are easily utilized by the body. A person who has not eaten for some time and takes a drink of alcohol energizes the body with this supply of calories. It can therefore function as a quick pick-me-up for the drinker. That reward is not quickly forgotten. Even after the alcohol has destroyed many areas of the alcoholic's life, he or she will relate the drinking experience to this pleasant initial aspect of drinking.

In addition to the calories provided by the alcohol, it has another property that produces initial stimulation. Alcohol lowers the inhibitions of the drinker. It depresses the functions of the brain that control judgment. Self-inflicted behavioral controls are negated by the alcohol. With fears and inhibitions reduced, there is a greater likelihood of social interaction. The normally shy individual receives some stimulating instant courage and performs in direct contrast to his or her normal personality. This inhibition reducer, combined with the quickly absorbed calories, gives alcohol its stimulating initial effect.

The last reason that alcohol has an initial stimulating effect is due to another unique property. What alcohol does to a person has a lot to do with what the person expects it to do. For instance, the same chemical that is relaxing to one person after a hard day of work is what energizes someone else to go and dance all evening. A drinker may find a beer tastes good and is relaxing with dinner. That same drinker may find beer to be the substance that produces yelling and screaming for the home team at a baseball game. Champagne might be consumed on a romantic evening alone or at a wedding reception and have two entirely different effects. The effect of alcohol is closely related to the mind-set of the drinker and the setting of its consumption.

All of these factors produce a chemical that can have opposite effects. Perhaps that is why it has fascinated people for centuries. It is also a reason that adolescents should not drink. At a time when their own behavior is often erratic and judgment is often poor, it is best that alcohol not be introduced to the various situations they face. Dating can result in disasters when teenagers are stimulated by alcohol at the same time as it reduces their inhibitions. Adolescence is a volatile time, and the alcohol only makes it more so. Teenagers need help in making good decisions, and alcohol does not help. For many adolescents, alcohol is neither a stimulant or a depressant; they drink, and drink fast, to the point of drunkenness. For them the myth is irrelevant. What alcohol is to them is a killer. And more teenagers will die from drunk driving than from any other cause—it is their number one killer. It is also the reason why life expectancy has increased in every age category, except for adolescents. If death is as far down as you get to go, then alcohol is the ultimate downer. It gets more kids to that point than anything else in the world.

In working with advanced alcoholics, it is very important to remember both the stimulating and the depressing effects of the alcohol. It helps to explain why people who are extremely depressed from too much alcohol will continue to go back to the bottle for relief. They crave the energizing, quick pick-me-up that comes from the calories and from satisfying the addiction by ingesting more of the addictive chemical. Because the nerve cells in the central nervous system crave the substance, nothing else will satisfy. The alcoholic's central nervous system functions at its peak when the alcohol is drunk. This makes alcohol a stimulus to the central nervous system because of the addiction factor. The physical dependency on the alcohol has far exceeded any psychological dependency that might have developed. Treatment is needed to assist the alcoholic in abandoning the alcohol and starting a new life. If support is not provided to encourage the alcoholic to continue, he or she will relapse back into drinking before recovery starts. The depression experienced in the acute withdrawal stage can be severe. If proper support is not there until the depression lifts, the alcoholic will return to the bottle for the stimulating effects of the chemical. If alcohol were only a downer, another drug could be used to provide relief.

2. *Alcohol affects everyone in the same manner.*

Every person's system is different, so that each varies in how fast the alcohol is metabolized and how quickly the intoxicating effects are felt. Tolerance is a key to how alcohol affects people. Someone with a very low tolerance will become very drunk, to the point of sickness or passing out, on a small amount of alcohol. A person with a high tolerance can drink unbelievable amounts of alcohol and not become intoxicated. It is hard for many to believe that some alcoholics can drink more than a case of beer and not be intoxicated.

Of course, weight is a factor in how alcohol affects a person. The heavier the person, the slower the action of alcohol, but the varying effects go beyond the weight factor. Two people weighing exactly the same will differ in how alcohol affects them. One may fall asleep on one beer, and the other may feel absolutely no effect. This is an essential concept for teenagers to know. They must understand that not being able to "hold your liquor" is not a sign of weakness. It is merely the result of a difference in the way alcohol is metabolized by different systems. If an adolescent drinks to keep up with the crowd, and the crowd has a much higher tolerance, passing-out drunkenness or illness will result. The person will be out of control. There is no value in being able to drink more than someone else. In fact, a high tolerance early in life is a warning sign that alcoholism may be developing.

Studies on the effects of alcohol show an apparent involvement of a hereditary factor. Marc A. Schuckit, M.D., professor of psychiatry at the University of California, San Diego School of Medicine, has studied the sons of alcoholics to determine differences in children of alcoholics and nonalcoholics. One study revealed that the sons of alcoholics tend to become *less* intoxicated with the consumption of higher amounts of alcohol. That being the case, children of alcoholics are born with the ability to drink more alcohol. This allows them to consume more of the addictive chemical and makes them more susceptible to the addiction process. Chapter Four examines the research indicating the hereditary component of alcoholism.

Interviewing and discussing drinking with alcoholics and nonalcoholics brings out marked differences in the experiences. The nonalcoholic relates a rather benign experience and displays a take-it-or-leave-it attitude; he or she may describe a drink as relaxing or a way to spend time with friends. But the alcoholic, when not in denial, relates a more emotional experience of drinking. Words like "warmth," "security," and "wholeness," are used—words someone else might use to describe the feelings of being with a best friend. No matter how severe the alcoholism, it seems that the alcoholic will talk in terms of what the alcohol used to do or the effects it used to produce. Perception and misperception play a large role in the effects of alcohol, and an alcoholic who is deluded by the addiction process cannot accurately describe the total effect of the chemical.

Alcohol's effect varies greatly among different drinkers. Blanket generalizations about its effects show a lack of insight into the properties of the chemical; its uniqueness comes from its widely varied effects. But for the alcoholic, one effect cannot be denied: addiction. That addiction pulls the alcoholic into drinking behavior that eventually results in devastation.

3. Alcohol is just another drug.

The preceding passage indicates that it isn't. Alcohol is a unique chemical that affects different people in different ways. A factor that significantly separates alcohol from other drugs is that it is *selectively* addictive. Some people—most people—cannot become addicted to alcohol. This statement is admittedly very controversial. On the surface it appears to be totally false, but looking beyond the obvious reveals the truth of alcohol's addictive powers.

Most people believe that if you drink enough alcohol long enough, you are certain to become an alcoholic. This is not true. First of all, alcohol is an addictive chemical. One drink does not have much addictive power. A couple of drinks are not going to drive a person into addiction. Most people have an automatic limiting mechanism that prevents them from drinking enough alcohol to become addicted.

Automatic limiting mechanisms come in different forms. Some people cannot drink a lot because of a low tolerance; a drink or two would cause severe intoxication and the inability to drink more. For others, passing out occurs after drinking very little. The limit is automatic, because you cannot drink if you are not awake. The other limiting mechanism is getting sick. A lot of drinkers cannot drink very much because they get sick and throw up after very little drinking. Alcohol must be consumed in larger quantities for it to addict the body. If it cannot be drunk in large amounts, addiction is automatically prevented.

Most people have and maintain a low tolerance throughout life. As they grow older, it gradually increases, but not significantly. You could make a case for most people becoming addicted if they drank long enough, but the rate at which the tolerance goes up would require living to age 165 or 190.

Alcohol's selectively addictive properties differ from those of a drug like heroin. Probably 95 percent of those who inject heroin become addicted; for some reason the other 5 percent do not, probably because of some adverse reaction to the heroin. But for most who inject heroin, there is no automatic limiting mechanism to prevent the addiction. It is exactly opposite from alcohol.

Alcoholics do not have the automatic limiting mechanism nonalcoholic drinkers do. They drink vast quantities of alcohol with little observable effect. Many maintain their alcohol level just below the point of intoxication. Although problems are not evident in the early drinking phase, they are developing below the observation level. Alcohol is addictive. A case of beer is a lot of addictive chemical, enough to cause significant withdrawal when the drinking stops. That withdrawal will drive the person to drink again.

About 80 percent of drinkers will not develop alcoholism or alcohol addiction, because they cannot. Their bodies will not allow enough of the drug to be consumed. Other drugs, like heroin, have a much higher rate of addictability, and most who use them over time will become addicted. Alcohol's selectively addictive properties separate it from other mood-altering drugs.

4. You cannot become an alcoholic on just beer or wine.

Alcohol is an addictive chemical. It does not matter what form it comes in. If you take pure alcohol and put it in oranges, then those oranges become addictive. Alcohol in a malt beverage or alcohol in a sweet drink topped off with a cute umbrella is equally addicting. What the alcohol is in is less important than how much is consumed. This myth is a common belief among alcoholics, and it is often accepted by their spouses. It is not unusual to hear an alcoholic say, "I'm not an alcoholic; I only drink beer," or "I can't be an alcoholic; I don't drink anything but wine."

Opinions differ on the indicators of heavy drinking. One measure of a heavy drinker is as follows: anyone who drinks five drinks or more at least three times a week. This level of drinking should be a warning sign to the drinker and the drinker's family. It is an indicator of a progressing alcohol problem. It does not matter what those drinks are. They can be twelve ounces of beer, four and one-half ounces of wine, or one and one-half ounces of eighty-proof spirits. The amount of alcohol is almost the same, and all are equally addicting in large quantities.

5. If you can control your drinking, you are not an alcoholic.

Loss of control has been a major indicator of alcoholism for centuries. Certainly if a person cannot control the consumption of alcohol, he or she is almost by definition an alcoholic, and well into the later stages. But the seemingly obvious corollary is not true: the ability to control the drinking does not prove that alcoholism is absent. It just means that alcoholism has not reached the later stages.

The fact is, people who are not alcoholic have no need to control their drinking. The alcoholic, as the alcoholism progresses, becomes increasingly obsessed with the ability to control the alcohol consumption. Few people question whether or not they are in control of the number of carrots they eat. They do not question it because it is not a problem. People try to control what is obviously a problem. If someone must continually make an effort to control drinking, it is a sign of alcoholism that has progressed at least to the middle stages.

This issue has caused some confusion in research on alcoholics and their ability to drink socially. What researchers observed was "controlled alcoholic drinking." Controlled alcoholic drinking occurs at a point of high motivation for an alcoholic. In a period of controlled drinking, an alcoholic is not presenting a problem; he or she may drink one or two drinks and no more. Researchers have called this a return to social drinking, but it is not. An alcoholic, totally focused on maintaining control, being sure that two or three drinks is the limit, is hardly drinking socially. It is only a matter of time before he or she loses control again. When the researchers are gone and the motivation is less, the uncontrolled drinking will continue again.

Some counselors, mental-health professionals, and physicians use tests to determine whether or not a person can control drinking. The questionable alcoholic is instructed to drink two shots of alcohol every day. The theory is that if someone can drink those two drinks and *only* those two drinks for a month, then alcoholism is not a problem. The ability to consume two drinks a day for a month means nothing. Probably the person is being instructed to take the test because someone close has demanded seeking the help of a professional. The test is not a test of alcoholism but a test of motivation.

A common occurrence in alcoholic families is for the spouse eventually to confront the alcoholic about drinking. The alcoholic, denying that drinking is a problem, will suggest a test or proof to verify that it isn't: "If I can go one month without drinking, will you believe that I do not have a problem?" Sure enough, for one month the alcoholic will "white-knuckle it" and not drink. It means nothing. There is better than a 90 percent chance that the person is an alcoholic. That type of test does not happen in families where there is no alcoholism. The ability to control drinking is just an indicator that alcoholism may still be in the early or middle stages.

MYTHS ABOUT ALCOHOLICS AND DRINKERS

6. *Alcoholics drink to relieve stress, tension, and anxiety. Everyone else, especially social drinkers, is just drinking to be sociable.*

Everyone drinks for the same reason. They may tell you they

drink because they like the taste. Or they may tell you they drink to be sociable. But people drink for the effect of the alcohol. If it were not for the effect, people would drink straight club soda. It is the social drinker who is drinking to relieve stress and tension. "Happy hours" (or unhappy hours) are filled with social drinkers who are drinking to relax and reduce the tension of the day. Alcoholics do the same in the early stages of their drinking. That motivation to drink or the reason for continual drinking changes for the alcoholic.

Eventually, the alcoholic who started drinking for the same reason as everyone else drinks for a different reason. The drinking is continued and increased to satisfy the growing power of addiction. Alcoholics drink to relieve the stress that everyone else experiences, but their stress is compounded by physiological deterioration, a result of the damage done to the system by the vast amounts of alcohol. This deterioration reduces the ability to cope. Since the nervous system is greatly irritated by the large doses of alcohol, minor stresses take a greater toll and produce a stronger agitation. The alcoholic's drinking relieves both physical and mental pain. The anguish differs vastly from the normal everyday stresses of nonalcoholics.

Alcoholics drink for two other reasons: for the stimulating effect and for enhanced performance. When the level of alcohol is reduced in the alcoholic's body, withdrawal begins. The new alcohol stops the withdrawal process and improves and maintains the performance of the alcoholic.

In the beginning, the alcoholic's motivation to drink is the same as everyone else's. But the reason for drinking changes, becoming the satisfaction of a very powerful addiction. When people tell the alcoholic that alcohol is the problem, he or she believes it is the answer: it is the only source of relief from the pain of withdrawal and the craving of the addiction.

7. People become alcoholics because they have some form of mental illness.

Alcoholism begins as a problem, with the body doing something with the alcohol that other bodies don't do. Rather than experiencing a predictable reaction that limits consumption, the alcoholic adapts to the chemical. As the adaptation continues, tolerance increases and addiction takes control of both the body and the mind. If you look at the result of alcoholism, you might think that alcoholics are crazy. Alcoholics do crazy things, but the craziness occurs because the alcohol has made the brain toxic. The toxicity destroys the brain's ability to function normally.

Before they develop alcoholic drinking patterns, alcoholics display no more and no fewer signs of mental illness than abstainers and social drinkers. The same is true for those who stop drinking. When recovery is complete, the craziness stops. The alcoholic's personality returns to normal—if that's what it was before. Of course, if the alcoholic was mentally ill before drinking, he or she will be mentally ill when the drinking stops.

There have been many attempts to pinpoint a specific mental condition that leads to alcoholism, but there is no such condition. Alcoholics have only one thing in common: the ability to drink a lot of alcohol. That difference is a physiological one, not a psychological difference. There is no preexisting mental illness common to alcoholics.

The concept of a predisposing mental illness is similar to the belief that alcoholism is caused by a spiritual problem. Alcoholism destroys a person's ability to grow spiritually. Much guilt and anger result from years of drinking and irrational behavior. The spiritual problem was not the cause, but the result. If recovery is to be complete, the spiritual dimension must be part of the solution. Spiritual problems are common among those with drinking problems, as is mental illness, neither should be confused with the source of the problem. The source is the alcoholic's body and how it metabolizes alcohol.

Why is this an important concept for the alcoholic to accept? In recovery, spiritual growth will occur and mental stability will return. If the alcoholic believes that spiritual or mental problems caused the alcoholic drinking, once these areas improve, the alcoholic will feel he or she has a license to drink "moderately" again. Understanding that alcoholism is physical helps with the acceptance of the need for total abstinence. The alcoholic will grow spiritually and mentally, but treatment will not provide a new body. The same body that did not drink normally before treatment will not drink normally after treatment. If an alcoholic does not accept that fact, he or she may try to grow spiritually or mentally to be able to drink again. No mental condition causes alcoholism. If the alcoholic can accept that, there is a greater chance for complete recovery. If friends and family can accept it and reinforce that, it will help the alcoholic in the recovery process.

8. The real person emerges under the influence of alcohol.

In vino veritas—in wine is truth—represents a misconception about alcohol's effect on people. Some think that character insights are revealed by what a person does when drunk.

Alcoholic drinking destroys the individual's ability to think rationally and feel appropriately. In effect, it produces a very sick personality. The alcoholic's personality is a distorted caricature of the original personality before the drinking. Eventually the drinking completely destroys the character of the alcoholic. In a struggle to survive, the alcoholic continues the destructive drinking.

Once the alcoholic is sober and the toxic effects of the chemical have worn off, the real person emerges. Those disgusting and irrational behaviors do not return. If they were the "real" person, they would surface from time to time. But they do not in the life of a truly recovering alcoholic. There is no "hidden" person that is revealed only by the effects of alcohol.

In recovery there is a lot of initial guilt and shame over what happened during the drinking. The alcoholic is committed to change, never to repeat the acts, to improve whatever personality is there. This is really the most important point about an alcoholic: not that the true person was evident in drunkenness, but that a real person can emerge in the recovery process. Alcoholics who recover have a phenomenal potential for change. That change into who the person will be is more important than what the person did while drinking.

9. Alcoholics have an addictive personality. This addictive personality is the real cause of the alcoholism.

The more accurate statement would be that an *addicted* personality exists. The original symptoms of alcoholism are invisible to most people, and to them it appears that an obsession with alcohol develops and compulsive drinking results. But that is not so. As the tolerance for alcohol increases, more alcohol is consumed, and the physical addiction grows more powerful and leads to a preoccupation or obsession with the chemical alcohol. An individual addicted to a chemical is not in control of drives or emotions. When the alcoholic attempts to control the drinking, the addiction drives him or her to do other things to excess, so eating, smoking, gambling, or like behaviors will increase. What appears to be a propensity to react in an addictive way is actually an addict grasping at anything that will reduce the emotional and physical pain from not being able to satisfy the addiction.

Once the addiction process is understood, it is easy to see the predictability of the behavior of the alcoholic. The alcoholic drinks compulsively because of the addiction. Then, reinforcing the denial of the problem, the alcoholic cuts down on the drinking to prove that control is being maintained. Extinguishing one compulsive behavior drives the person to other compulsive behaviors. This syndrome is the basis for the "addictive personality."

One common observation of alcoholics is that many quit drinking alcohol and instead drink gallons of coffee and smoke cartons of cigarettes, which reinforces the belief that there is an addictive personality at the base of the problem. The truth is that the compulsive coffee drinker and chain-smoker is not completely recovered from alcoholism. Quality recovery is free of compulsive behavior and addictive chemicals of all types. This is not to condemn those who still drink a lot of coffee and smoke a lot of cigarettes; it is just to say that there is further room for growth. More areas need to be resolved. Then what appears to be an addictive personality will become a revived and restored personality.

10. Adolescents are too young to be alcoholics. They may have some problems that involve alcohol, but alcoholism would be an inaccurate diagnosis.

Listen to a sixteen-year-old talk about filling her thermos with vodka to drink during lunch and you start to believe that adolescents can be alcoholics. Some adolescents become physically addicted to alcohol. They find themselves unable to live without a drink. Their whole attention is focused on the time and place of the next drink.

Age is not a factor when it comes to alcoholism. If a person has a predisposition toward alcoholism and that person drinks, it is only a matter of time until the obvious symptoms of alcoholism surface. Age is important in one way: It appears that the younger a person starts drinking, the faster alcoholism develops.

The drinking clock seems to work much faster in those who drink very young; the progression that might span twenty years will be played out in less than three years in an adolescent's life. The point of losing total control of drinking comes very early for many teenagers.

Many adolescents experience problem drinking. They get intoxicated frequently and will have some alcohol-related problems. Most teenagers grow out of that stage. They stop the repeated drunkenness and lower their frequency of drinking. Some do not grow out of it; they are saddled with an addiction to the chemical. They are in need of more than help from a psychologist specializing in adolescent problems; they need treatment in an alcoholism treatment center.

11. Alcoholics can return to social drinking once the sources of internal conflict are identified and resolved.

The experience of thousands of alcoholics demonstrates that this is not true. Time and again alcoholics relapse and return to treatment because they attempted to drink socially. An alcoholic may control the drinking for a short length of time, but social drinking is not a possibility for the recovering alcoholic. Most likely the alcoholic never drank socially at any time in his or her drinking. It is a waste of time for the alcoholic to attempt social drinking. The effort needs to be spent on establishing a solid program for total recovery. That recovery program calls for complete honesty. The alcoholic who is completely honest knows that social drinking will never be a reality. The faulty drinking body system will remain faulty for a lifetime.

MYTHS ABOUT ALCOHOLISM

12. Alcoholism is a secondary problem. There is a deeper problem that is primary and must be resolved.

For a long time some psychiatrists and psychologists have been frustrated in working with alcoholics. Once or twice a week they try to help the alcoholic gain "insight" into the problem—the deeper problem—from which the alcoholism is supposedly manifested. They approach this problem from many theoretical bases. Some use relaxation therapy, some use hypnotism, and some use psychoanalysis. Many other methods are used to help the alcoholic gain a deeper understanding and realization of what lies beneath the drinking. But these methods do not help the alcoholic. They may produce some short-term results, but ultimately they are merely postponing long-term recovery.

Alcoholics need treatment. That treatment process will help the person stop drinking and start dealing with the reality of today. Treatment is not a means by which alcoholics learn insight into their past. Today, and how to live it sober, is the priority. Put enough "todays" together and you come up with weeks and months without alcohol. The body and the mind free themselves from toxic chemicals. Thinking and emotions return to normal. As time goes on, some insight develops. But that insight does not focus on some preexisting personality disorder or a mental handicap. The insight comes from the realization that the alcoholic's drinking is different from that of other people who drink socially. It either was different from the beginning or it developed into a different pattern. The alcoholic gains further insight when he or she realizes that the drinking will never be like other people's drinking. It is useless to try over and over again to make it appear normal; the only route is to achieve total abstinence, one day at a time.

Psychological and psychiatric guidance can be utilized to help the alcoholic deal with the emotion that produces most relapses: guilt. Because the drinking has caused so much irrational behavior, and those actions have hurt others, the alcoholic is usually saddled with a tremendous amount of guilt. If the alcoholic does not resolve the guilt, he or she will return to drinking to find relief from it. Help from mental-health professionals is crucial. It is done on the other side of treatment. It must occur after the person has stopped drinking. It is the only kind of "insight" therapy that is helpful to the alcoholic.

Alcoholism is a problem unto itself that must be treated according to the way that millions have been successfully treated. The alcoholic must gain insight into the value of those treatments. Society must erase its ignorance with insight into how alcoholics can best maintain sobriety. Searching for an underlying cause is a waste of time. There is no common predrinking condition that produces alcoholism. There are no collective personality traits that make a person alcoholic. Alcoholics do not differ from nonalcoholics socially, psychologically, normally, spiritually, or mentally at the onset of drinking. They do differ physiologically. The body adapts to the chemical, tolerance goes up, and addiction traps the person into a life-style of futile attempts at self-treatment and coping. Recovery comes, not from insight, but from the realization that help, support, and direction are needed in developing a life-style free from alcohol.

13. Alcoholism is a moral problem that needs a spiritual solution.

The spiritual aspects of recovery should never be minimized. It is a difficult concept to understand and prevents many alcoholics from joining a group that professes to acknowledge God. Allowing God to help in areas where we have been helpless is important for recovery. Searching for truth that leads to a knowledge of a divine God who is for us and not against us is vital for the truly recovering alcoholic. It is sad to see sobriety and recovery attempted without God. It leads to a poor quality of life, continued alienation, and lingering guilt feelings. The guilt feelings have much to do with the importance of spiritual recovery. The irresponsible and immoral acts committed while drinking must be resolved. This part of spiritual recovery has to do with accepting forgiveness for those acts, feeling forgiven, and forgiving yourself. The spiritual aspect of recovery is vital for long-term sobriety.

It is not the only dimension of recovery, though, because alcoholism is not a moral problem. Many alcoholics under the influence or experiencing withdrawal say and do immoral things. Those immoral things come out of a brain saturated with a chemical that is both addictive and toxic. Alcoholics are not in full control of either their emotions or thoughts, and their actions are grossly distorted from their predrinking condition. The physical dimension must be a priority; the alcoholic must be physically detoxified from the chemical and nutritionally built up to regain strength and heal damaged nerve tissue. In the mental dimension, new information must be imparted during recovery: what alcoholism is and why it develops. The alcoholic will understand that he or she is not alone, that the actions and reactions were a predictable part of the progression of the disease. Psychologically, the alcoholic needs to resolve some emotions and learn to express and manage feelings appropriately. Socially, new friends and new activities need to be incorporated into everyday living. Positive and supportive people and places need to replace the negative and destructive. Each dimension— spiritual, social, physical, mental, and psychological—must be addressed and combined to form a system of recovery that produces long-term sobriety.

All of these areas are ruinously affected by alcoholism, and the ruin must be repaired in recovery. At times the clergy will focus on the spiritual area alone. They will try to convince people that it holds the key to the alcoholic's recovery. We repeat that it is vital, but it is not an isolated dimension. Professionals in other areas also want to focus on a single dimension. Nutritionists want to believe that changing what the alcoholic eats will produce sobriety; physical therapists might believe that exercise holds the key; the social worker may suggest that a new environment is the only hope for the alcoholic. All views hold some truth, taken together, but alone, they offer only temporary success and false hopes.

The moral question is such a major focus because of the nature of the problem. Before it is arrested, alcoholism destroys a person's judgment; immorality frequently results, and the result is seen as the cause. These immoral end products did not start the problem; society must not be fooled by what is seen on the surface after years of drinking.

Finally, the morality of the recovering alcoholic changes dramatically. The alcoholic develops a spiritual perspective and establishes priorities that are helpful, not harmful. Using people is replaced with serving people. Of course, not all recovering alcoholics reach this level of maturity. For them, recovery remains incomplete. The important point to note is that when all the dimensions of recovery are successfully addressed, a morally superior person emerges who is tremendously different from the drinking or practicing alcoholic. If there were a moral root to the problem before the drinking, it would remain after the drinking stopped. But it does not. Morals, as well as every other dimension of the alcoholic, change during the recovery process.

14. Alcoholism can be defined as a condition that exists when alcohol affects any aspect of a person's life: physical, mental, emotional, social, or spiritual.

If alcohol affects any one of these aspects, it is an indication that drinking has become a problem. By that time, in most cases, the alcoholism has progressed into the middle and late stages.

Each aspect can be subdivided into areas: financial, family, school, or job. Usually the problem shows up last at work. By the time the drinking has become so uncontrollable that work is affected, most of the other areas, especially the family, have been devastated by the progressing problem.

Education and increased knowledge will allow society to detect alcohol problems before they reach the point of destroying the alcoholic and the alcoholic's family. It must be recognized that the key identifying factor of alcoholism is the ability to drink an excessive amount of alcohol. Drinking a lot of an addictive chemical will produce addiction; the results of the addiction may show up early or late, but they will always emerge. People who drink a lot must not be enabled to continue by passing it off as "being able to hold my liquor." The drinking must be identified and confronted as harmful to the individual, the family, and society at large. When we begin recognizing and intervening in drinking problems early, we will save people from emotional destruction as well as saving the millions of dollars and tens of thousands of lives that alcoholism costs this nation each year. Alcoholism is more than just hampered performance in one of life's dimensions; it is addiction to alcohol, which begins with a growing tolerance to the chemical. That tolerance, admired by some, is at the heart of the alcoholism problem. Most people will never develop a high tolerance to the chemical and will never be addicted to it.

It is important to clarify the difference between alcoholism and problem drinking. Whereas alcoholism will afflict about 20 percent of people who drink, problem drinking can happen to anyone who drinks. Problem drinking occurs when a person drinks beyond the tolerance level and becomes drunk. That drunkenness leads to loss of control; the loss of control causes drunk driving, unintended sexual activity, violence, and many other too familiar difficulties. So plenty of people who are not alcoholics, who are not developing an alcohol addiction, can be irresponsible and have an alcohol problem. These problem drinkers are the ones who can be helped by some form of insight therapy. They do need help before they kill or hurt themselves or someone else while driving drunk.

A lot of teenagers are problem drinkers. Many college students indulge in problem drinking on weekends. Most, if they survive, grow out of this phase. They mature and no longer drink to the point of intoxication. Some do not grow out of the problem. They are unable to change because their bodies adapt to the chemical and become dependent on it. For these alcoholics, problem or irresponsible drinking is just the beginning.

Many alcoholics do not drink in an observable problem-drinking pattern. If the tolerance is so high that the alcoholic is drunk on twelve beers, and only ten beers are consumed, then drunkenness will not result and problem drinking will not be evident. Problem drinking for the alcoholic may be rare if most of the drinking is done below the limit level. Many alcoholics avoid repeated intoxication until the late stages of alcoholism, when tolerance often drops dramatically and drinking becomes uncontrollable. With greater knowledge, progressing alcoholism could be identified with high tolerance.

Alcoholism and problem drinking, though distinctly different, are usually confused. The distinction allows for appropriate treatment for both types of problems as early as possible.

15. There are many different types of alcoholism.

There is only one type of alcoholism. The myth arises from the various stages of alcoholism. What appears to be a special type of alcoholism is alcoholism that has stagnated in a particular stage. People vary in how quickly they progress through the stages. For some the progression happens over months, and for some it takes years, but it is the same problem. No matter how fast or slow the progression, it always results in uncontrollable drinking. The need is to identify the alcoholism before it reaches the uncontrollable-drinking phase.

16. Alcoholism is a slow form of suicide.

Alcoholism is not a means by which the alcoholic *chooses* to die. In the late stages of alcoholism, the alcoholic is beyond the point of choice. He or she is trapped in the addiction process. Unless someone intervenes, there is not much hope for recovery.

If an alcoholic in the late stages wanted to die, the quickest way would be to stop drinking. Withdrawal, or delirium tremens (d.t.'s), does kill alcoholics. The alcoholic who wants to stop drinking may have to start again to prevent withdrawal from resulting in seizures or death. So instead of alcoholism being a slow form of suicide by choice, it is a miserable form of survival by necessity. The proof is in the thousands who have hit bottom, lost everything, and miraculously recovered. Once an alcoholic is given the alternative of recovery and the support and motivation needed for sobriety, he or she will most often abandon the progression toward death.

17. Drunkenness is an indicator of alcoholism.

As mentioned earlier, drunkenness is an indicator of irresponsible and problem drinking, not necessarily of alcoholism. Many alcoholics drink for years without repeatedly becoming intoxicated. In many cases the drunkenness happens late in the progression. It should never serve as the only indication of an alcohol problem. Many other signs can precede drunkenness. The principal symptom is a high tolerance for alcohol.

18. Moderate drinking is the key to avoiding alcoholism.

For many people, the only way to avoid alcoholism is to not drink at all. If a person is born with a predisposition toward alcoholism and then drinks, alcoholism will progress whether or not that person tries to maintain a moderate drinking level.

An alcoholic can sometimes drink moderately, for many reasons. Motivation is usually the biggest factor. For instance, an alcoholic man wanting to impress his future bride might use all of his will to control his drinking at a moderate level. But once married, his motivation may lower, and the moderate drinking may turn into uncontrollable drinking. No matter how much willpower and motivation are used to moderate the drinking, the addiction will always be stronger; it will overpower the person and destroy the attempts to drink moderately. If effort is needed to drink in a responsible or moderate manner, that is a key indicator that alcoholism is present, not that it has been avoided.

19. Alcoholic progression is always a slow process.

The clock for the progression of the alcoholism varies for each person. One guarantee of speeding up that clock is to drink early in life. Some kids have progressed to the later stages of alcoholism by the time they reach the age of twelve or thirteen. Adolescent alcoholics verify that the entire journey through the stages of alcoholism can be a quick one. On the other hand, some develop no late-stage symptoms until past the age of eighty.

Whether progression is fast or slow, it is vital that alcoholism be recognized and confronted at the earliest possible stage.

20. Alcoholism is not a disease. It is a temporary problem that most people outgrow.

Many people hate to hear alcoholism referred to as a disease. They are afraid that if the alcoholic thinks that it is a disease, he or she will not accept responsibility for the problem. Whether or not an alcoholic accepts responsibility for the problem is not important. What is important is for the alcoholic to accept responsibility for recovery. Part of that responsibility involves making amends for things done in the past. That is the essential thing, not assigning or accepting blame.

Alcoholics need to be able to accept alcoholism as a disease. It is an essential part of the recovery process. The alcoholic must not believe that in time, alcoholism will be outgrown; it must be viewed as a disease that can be arrested but not cured. It is a disease because it has identifiable symptoms that affect the individual in a predictable progression. The disease is chronic, progressive, and potentially fatal. It is further manifested in the form of increased tolerance and physical dependency. The disease pathologically changes certain organs as it progresses.

It really does not matter what you call alcoholism. The important thing is that if you have it, you do something about it. There is value in labeling the problem as a disease, because just as this disease has easily identifiable symptoms, it also has specific treatments that will successfully arrest its progression. The uniqueness of the disease is that a physician alone cannot treat it. It takes a multidisciplinary approach. Once treatment is accepted, the alcoholic never needs to experience the symptoms of the disease again. Those alcoholics who do not accept treatment die twelve to fourteen years earlier than those who do not have the disease.

MYTHS ABOUT RECOVERY

21. If you know someone who is an alcoholic, the goal should be to help that person stop drinking.

The goal is not to get the alcoholic to stop drinking. The goal must be to help the alcoholic obtain treatment and start recovery. In fact, most alcoholics stop drinking many times before they finally recover. If the alcoholic is in denial, he or she will use the ability to stop as evidence that the drinking is still under control.

If people around the alcoholic plead for the alcoholic to stop drinking as a better way to live, the effort can produce the exact opposite outcome. The alcoholic may be so addicted that the body and mind function better when drinking than when not. If this is true, the alcoholic will feel more miserable without the alcohol during withdrawal. This will convince the alcoholic that, although alcohol was identified as the problem, he or she finds it a part of the solution. The improved performance when the drinking resumes reinforces this belief.

But if the goal is to get the alcoholic to treatment, the outcome is far different. With treatment there is strong support for recovery. The withdrawal stage can be managed medically and professionally. The strong denial of the alcoholic can be confronted. The entire treatment team and other recovering alcoholics in treatment will reinforce the recovery process and life-style change daily. With this approach, there is a much greater chance for long-term sobriety than with simply stopping drinking.

22. *Alcoholics can stop drinking on their own if they want to.*

Most alcoholics, except those in the late stages, can stop drinking on their own. The problem is *staying* stopped, which is rarely possible. In any case, stopping drinking alone will not improve the quality of life.

Some alcoholics are so addicted that it is impossible for them to stop permanently. When the flow of alcohol is cut off, withdrawal discomfort becomes so intense that the prospects of death or insanity appear very real, and fear of them drives the alcoholic back to the bottle again. The other motivation for a return to alcohol is the extreme guilt that the alcoholic feels. Looking at a devastated past, the guilt becomes overwhelming, until quick relief from the guilt comes with another drink.

Many people make the mistake of expecting the alcoholic to recover alone. They expect an instantaneous flash of insight that produces a life-style free of alcohol. Although in some rare cases this has happened, it is not very likely. The more realistic and successful approach is to assist the alcoholic in seeking treatment.

23. An alcoholic must lose everything before being helped.

This is an old belief based on early experience with recovering alcoholics. Before intervention techniques and treatment were widely known and available, losing absolutely everything was the only way that people recovered. The problem with this approach is one of motivation. Motivation for recovery is much higher when the alcoholic still has a job, family, and other support systems.

The goal must be to help the alcoholic as early in the progression as possible. It is irresponsible to sit back and watch the disease progress without intervening. No one would do that if the person had a different type of illness, like cancer or heart disease. Early intervention saves lives. It saves the lives of alcoholics and the significant others who are also affected by the progression of the problem.

24. An alcoholic must want help before being helped.

Most alcoholics who receive help today are coerced and even forced into treatment. Once there, it is the job of the treatment team to change the motivation from meeting demands to wanting a better life. The alcoholic is addicted to the chemical and is battling the effects of addiction or withdrawal. In addition, the alcohol is a mood-altering chemical, distorting reality and preventing the person from dealing appropriately with the problem. Denial is so strong that many alcoholics are paralyzed and cannot do what needs to be done to resolve the problem. The alcoholic will likely see drinking as a solution to the situation. What is obvious to others remains hidden from the alcoholic. Do not wait for the alcoholic to want help; the person's delusional world prevents him or her from taking constructive action toward solving the problem.

25. It is important to find out why an alcoholic drinks.

Countless alcoholics know exactly why they drink, but they continue to drink. There is no value in knowing the reasons behind the drinking. The reasons change from early drinking to late drinking. This myth arises from the belief that alcoholism has a psychological rather than a physiological base. Many people are recovering from alcoholism who have never stopped to consider the ''whys'' behind the drinking. It is more important

to know how to live one day at a time than it is to know why
drinking has continued over the years.

26. *Psychotherapy can help an alcoholic stop drinking and
achieve sobriety.*

Psychotherapy is not helpful to a person who is drunk six
days a week and sober one day, the day of therapy. The alcoholic
must stop drinking first and start recovering; then a therapist
can help in developing an understanding of the reactions of family and friends to the progression of alcoholism. The therapist
can be a strong source of accountability that will make the recovery strong and stable. The therapist can also be a valuable
resource in helping the alcoholic express new emotions.

27. *A sedative or tranquilizing drug is a healthy way to stop
drinking.*

Nothing could be further from the truth. Another mood-
altering chemical will only develop a dual addiction as the
alcoholic becomes cross-addicted. Valium does not resolve personal problems or treat the family. All it does is prevent recovery. It certainly does not help the alcoholic build character. Its
only value comes during detoxification process when used to
ease the withdrawal process.

Eventually the alcoholic will forsake the tranquilizer for the
alcohol, because Valium is inferior to alcohol as a mood-altering
chemical. Valium does not have the supply of calories for the
initial stimulation that alcohol provides and is merely a downer
drug.

Alcoholics must learn to delay gratification. The tranquilizer
continues to function as a short-term answer rather than a long-
term solution. The alcoholic must also learn to deal with reality.
The tranquilizer only distorts reality and distracts the alcoholic's
perception of the world. It is disastrous for anyone to suggest
that an alcoholic attempt to resolve the problem with a tranquilizer or sedative drug.

28. *Alcoholics Anonymous helps the drinker reach the maturity
level of nondrinkers and social drinkers.*

Social drinkers often drink to ease the stress and tension of
everyday life, but recovering alcoholics, who must remain abstinent, do not have the option of seeking an external means of

easing stress and tension. Each alcoholic must learn to cope with stress and anxiety free of alcohol and drugs. In addition, the alcoholic must stay sober and cope with stress with a central nervous system that has been damaged by saturation with alcohol and subsequent withdrawal. Further, after going through treatment, the alcoholic has come to see clearly all the devastation his or her drinking has caused, a realization that many social drinkers can avoid. Treatment has confronted the alcoholic with all his or her failures, mistakes, and missed opportunities. The alcoholic must deal with normal pressures and with all the dismaying reality of the past drinking years, and do it free of chemicals that are available to the social drinker. For that reason, alcoholics must *surpass* the level of maturity of nondrinkers and social drinkers. AA builds character and provides support and strength to enhance that process. In my experience, when recovery is complete, the level of maturity of the alcoholic exceeds that of people who have not suffered from the disease of alcoholism.

29. *Relapse is an indication of failure in the process of staying sober.*

Relapse is a predictable part of the disease of alcoholism. When a second heart attack occurs, we consider it just a part of heart disease. So why view relapse as failure rather than just a part of alcoholism? Relapse can be a true beginning point. It is an educational experience that says more honesty and support are needed to maintain sobriety. The key concept to remember is that of intervention in the relapse as soon as possible. The relapsed alcoholic will feel intense guilt and shame over returning to the booze. Act positive and reassure the person that no one has given up. Reinforce the commitment to treatment and reestablish the support system so that recovery may be long-term. The reaction to relapse has a greater impact on the alcoholic than the relapse itself. If the reactions are direct, caring, and supportive, the relapse can be a learning experience that begins the long-term recovery process.

30. *A recovering alcoholic is someone who has stopped drinking.*

An alcoholic may stop drinking and not be recovering. Stopping the drinking may produce symptoms worse than the drinking: overwhelming anger, guilt, and depression. For recovery to occur, the alcoholic must take steps to improve the quality of every dimension of life. Recovering alcoholics restore relationships and learn to share feelings. They become better employees, because they want to make an honest contribution and be productive. Recovering alcoholics do not go where they used to go or spend time with people they used to spend time with. They think and feel differently about themselves and others. They take care of their bodies. They eat nutritiously and exercise regularly. God is allowed to handle the parts of their lives that they cannot.

The recovering alcoholic is remarkably different from when he or she was drinking. His or her life exudes a natural and attractive serenity. In fact, when you are around a recovering alcoholic who has an enhanced quality of life, you are motivated to change your own life. You see the potential in yourself and others through the example of change in the recovering alcoholic. All over the world, men and women have stopped drinking and never started the recovery process. For them, life is an empty struggle to survive. They are not recovering from alcoholism.

In conclusion, the myths about alcoholism are numerous. These are but a few of those that cause the most problems. Don't be surprised to find that most of what is presented here directly contradicts what most people believe about the problem. That is exactly why we have so many hurt by alcoholism and a society that reacts only after the progression has taken a major toll on many lives. When thinking changes, more people will be spared the agony of suffering from alcoholism and not knowing what to do in time, or doing nothing because of the stigma associated with alcohol problems. The erasure of that stigma is the purpose of the material in this chapter. It can provide freedom to act, freedom to recover, and freedom to live again.

CHAPTER SIX

THE CODEPENDENT FAMILY OF ADDICTION

When addiction hits a family, it hits every member. No one is immune to its impact. It sweeps through family relationships like a flooding river from a broken dam. In its wake it leaves a devastated wasteland of guilt, fear, and anger. Nothing can so completely destroy a family as addiction. Whether it is addiction to alcohol, heroin, cocaine, or some other chemical, the results are the same: addiction wastes money, lives, potential, and entire families. If you have any uncertainty about that, talk to a family that has had a member addicted to a chemical. They are the proof that addiction never develops alone; it comes in families.

When I began working with alcoholics, the family dynamic was very clear early in my experience. I will never forget the first time I was confronted with the fact that there is more than a chemical involved in addiction. One case in particular stands out in my mind as showing what role the family plays and how addiction keeps people stuck in unhealthy roles. The case involved a man about age sixty-five and his wife of thirty years. The man had been a heavy drinker for most of his life and, like many alcoholics, spent a lot of time drinking without getting drunk very often. When he reached the age of forty-five, all that changed. His tolerance dropped and his drinking, along with the rest of his life, went completely out of control. He spent twenty years with an incredible drinking problem. His company gave him an early retirement, and for the last ten years his drinking had been extremely excessive. He was a very sick man by the time he came to us for help. He had seen his physician because of a very painful case of pancreatitis. The physician also diagnosed a severe case of cirrhosis of the liver. All he did was tell the man to check into our hospital. He agreed without hesitation and he came to the hospital that evening, escorted by his wife.

His wife had stood by him during the many years of drinking. She had called into work for him when he was too drunk or hung over to go. She would buy him more booze whenever he requested and was too sick to get out of bed. She lied for him, covered up for him, and remained faithful to him throughout the marriage. She had been a "saint," putting up with him for her entire life. Finally, it appeared that her dedication had paid off; he was entering treatment. She escorted him back to his room, waited until he was comfortably in bed, and kissed him good-bye. Then she went home, went to bed, and never woke up again. Incredible as it sounds, at the point at which his life began, hers ended. She died the very night he finally accepted help for the problem.

That is not the end of the story. The family came to the hospital the next day to tell their father the news. He wept all day. I expected him to leave treatment immediately and get himself drunk. But he did not leave. He stayed and completed treatment. And for as long as I kept in touch with him, he never drank again. If he is alive today, I imagine he is sober. But why did he depend on his wife to allow him to continue to drink? Why did she need a sick husband to take care of? It all has to do with the roles that trap the alcoholic and his or her family into codependency. If untreated, the family remains stuck in destructive roles which do not help the addict and which destroy each family member.

Another couple I met a few years ago exemplify the power that addiction and codependency hold over a married couple and a family. This case involved a female drug addict who was addicted to both tranquilizers and sleeping pills. She was, quite frankly, a mess when she came to us. Her whole appearance was deeply depressed. She was fat and apparently very miserable. She would take Librium, a tranquilizer, all day and then swallow a handful of sleeping pills at night. She was deeply addicted to both. She came to us after she tried to stop taking the pills on her own. When she did, she experienced violent hallucinations and went into withdrawal. Her husband brought her to us when he thought she was about to die. If he had not, she probably would have.

I remember that the detoxification process was a very long one for her. She had to have close supervision night and day for about five days. She was as sick as anyone I had ever seen coming off a drug of any kind. Finally, she was able to function in reality once again. But her struggle was not over after her first week. She was angry and bitter and wanted to leave treatment almost every day. Her system continued to adjust for the next six weeks. Little by little she gradually improved. She was a fighter, and eventually the fight went in her favor. She was determined to never touch another mood-altering chemical again. She knew that if she drank or took any other drug, it would be only a matter of time before she was back on her old medications.

This woman became very involved in the aftercare program at the hospital. She also volunteered many hours to help fellow addicts get help. As time went by, we were all amazed at her wonderful recovery. That year she lost over fifty pounds. She was undoubtedly one of the most transformed creatures I had ever seen. It was a fantastic year for her. She lived life to the fullest. On her one-year anniversary, or sobriety birthday, she attended a Narcotics Anonymous meeting and celebrated one year without alcohol and prescription drugs. To her it was the greatest accomplishment in her life. After the meeting, her husband took her out to eat to help her celebrate. When they arrived at the table, there was an already opened bottle of cold, bubbly champagne. Her glass was poured and waiting for her. Her husband, seeing her look of shock, told her that she deserved it; that it had been a great year. He had done this as a special reward to her for such a fabulous year. Fortunately, she turned around, walked out, took a cab, and came to the hospital to talk about what had happened.

Why did her husband do it? Why did he want to jeopardize her sobriety? Knowing how important her abstinence was, why would he ''reward'' her with alcohol? Of course, the answer was simple. Sad, but simple. She had done all the changing; he had not. He felt more insecure as her security increased. He wanted a helpless doormat back, but he did not get it. She, unlike many other addicts, did not fall prey to her sick husband's unconscious motives. He probably had no idea what he was actually doing. Since she was so healthy, she had no trouble seeing it. That marriage ended in divorce, a casualty of code-pendency.

It would be misleading to relate only these two negative stories. Here is one that shows the tremendous capacity to change—not just a person but an entire family. And especially a very stubborn husband.

A couple of months ago I received a phone call from a man I had met at the hospital about seven years earlier. His wife was undergoing treatment for drug addiction at the time. She had been using street drugs for years. Finally, when she became pregnant, her husband said he'd had enough. He literally dragged her to the hospital and told us we had to get her well. He was a stubborn, rigid, macho Texan who thought he had no problems. He considered himself a saint for having stayed with his wife through years of drug use. He could have been called a therapist's nightmare, because he was very difficult to work with. No one gave either him or his wife much hope for change. She was very sick, and he was tyrannical in his rule over her and their children. He trusted no one and wanted no part of counseling or counselors. His problems were his business and no one else's. Even bringing his wife to treatment had, to him, been a sign of weakness. In a case like that, where the person is so rigidly entrenched in a role, there is very little chance for change. The prognosis for her being allowed to recover fully and him adjusting healthily was guarded at best.

The phone call I received proved that no one can accurately predict who will change and who will get well. This stubborn, egotistical construction worker called me from the seminary that I had attended in Fort Worth, Texas. His life had changed dramatically and he was preparing to be a minister. He was preaching on the weekends, and his wife, the former drug addict, was an organist at the church. It was a very pleasant surprise to hear from him. It served as an excellent example of how people and families can change. In the worst of times there is always hope for a wonderful future.

For that hope to be realized, the members of an addicted family must break out of old, unhealthy behaviors and roles. These roles are destructive to the addict and the others in the addict's family. Each role can be adopted by any member of the family, and has its own unique behaviors that allow the addict to be addicted and the family member to survive in the symbiosis of codependency.

CHIEF ENABLER

Enabling is any behavior that allows the addict to continue to abuse without experiencing the full consequences of his or her behavior. It prevents the addict from achieving sobriety or entering the recovery process. Enabling allows the addict to deny the severity of the problem. To achieve this, a parent will ask a child to apologize to the addict for something that someone else was responsible for. A parent might lie to a schoolteacher about an illness when work is incomplete in an effort to cover up for a child who is a habitual pot smoker, unmotivated in school. A boss might enable an employee by doing some of his or her subordinate's work rather than take steps to correct the problem. Enabling is best described as doing all the wrong things for the right reasons. Because of care, concern, love, and a desire to help, people engage in all sorts of enabling behaviors. Rather than helping, they are allowing the addict to become sicker and the addiction to progress to the late stages.

The chief enabler is the person who is closest to the addict, the person who has the greatest ability to manipulate the environment around the addict. The goal of the chief enabler is to remove pain from the addict. To do that, the chief enabler will deny, lie, make excuses, and arrange to cover up every problem resulting from drinking. The pain that is lessened may be the one thing that could motivate the addict to accept treatment. That is why enabling is so destructive.

The chief enabler is often the addict's spouse. A wife might make excuses for her husband, saying he is out of town, sick, or busy when he is drunk or hung over. But it is not always the spouse. Parents often write off drug abuse as a stage or whim; they convince themselves it is just part of growing up. Husbands and wives may hide their child's addiction from each other or ignore the evidence that it exists. A son could even be a chief enabler to a father; he could drive him to the bar, pick him up, and lie to his mother about his time with Dad. Anyone can take on the chief enabler role. It is hard to give up.

The chief enabler role is clung to so strongly because it represents control, power, and often respect. There are some secondary benefits to being labeled the one without the problem. The chief enabler is viewed as a saint or a martyr. He or she is looked upon as a dedicated, loving spouse who has sacrificed everything for the addict. Respect from the children is almost guaranteed. By contrast to the other parent, the enabler stands head and shoulders above the addict, and having control of finances and every other area of the home can be a powerful inducement to continue to enable. If the addict is to get well, someone must show the chief enabler that there are some alternate behaviors available and that everyone can be free once the addict begins to recover. Rather than maintain a sick status quo, the chief enabler must be shown how to change the situation and motivate the addict and all the family to obtain help. If change is to occur, it is often the chief enabler who must initiate that change.

SUPERACHIEVER/FAMILY HERO

No one likes to be a part of a losing outfit. It is human nature to want to be a part of a winner. If you are in an organization, you want to be proud of it. You certainly do not want to be a member of something that is an embarrassment to you. It is particularly true that people do not want to be a part of a family that is failing. Most children will do anything to keep two parents together or to make the family at least look like a winner. It is out of this motivation that a family hero emerges to save the family name. This child, driven with a desire to excel, becomes a superachiever and outdistances family and friends in work and school. He or she wants to make the family a source of pride and give each member a good dose of self-worth. He or she is the caretaker of the family and will do anything to help the family survive.

The family hero believes that survival of the family depends on the addict's and the chief enabler's ability to continue in their roles. He or she is unaware of the option for both of these people to change, so the superachiever has the double task of supporting both the addict and the chief enabler. This is not an easy chore. It involves a lot of self-sacrifice and manipulation; it requires relentless determination to make things okay. This drive and the attitude of responsibility translate into an ability to get things done outside the family. The hero, through daily practice, learns to achieve and succeed, especially when persistence is required.

Those who observe superachieving family heroes see an outward success. They appear to always be willing to do what is right. They are able to live independently from the rest of the family. They are the picture of what it is to be a responsible person. If anyone "has it together," the superachievers seem to. But on the inside, they are a picture of emotional turmoil. They may look successful, but they feel inadequate and worth little. Their best never seems to be good enough. They are hurting and confused over the struggle in which they participate. Fear and loneliness push away the possibility of happiness. Often at the peak of a career or the height of recognition, the family hero collapses in an emotional breakdown or suffers from a severe illness. Many even commit suicide. Theirs is a world of constant struggle.

The driven superachiever/family hero is usually found at the top of the ranks in any area of accomplishment. He or she is driven into positions such as class president, team captain, valedictorian, corporate executive, or social leader. Now, none of these is wrong to do or achieve. But the family hero does not make the choice. He or she is driven, not choosing, to fill these roles.

Without help, superachievers/family heroes grow up to fill classic roles of workaholics and society saviors. They achieve status in many helping professions such as medicine, education, and even politics. All their lives they learn to make things happen and succeed independently; therefore, they are the least likely in the family to seek outside help. The toughest to work with in therapy or treatment, they are the most resistant to anyone knowing what is really going on inside. Often, while an entire family recovers, the family hero will continue in the struggle to find worth beyond the limitations of a family with a problem. It is no small task to help this person see the options and turn off the drive and the march toward achievement.

With help, family heroes can make some wonderful changes. Rather than feeling responsible for everything and everybody, these people are able to relax and accept responsibility for self. Rather than denying that they are ever wrong, they are able to accept failure as a part of life. The balance that can be produced when they obtain help allows them to be excellent employees.

Their personal lives experience a new freedom also; they are not driven to marry someone who needs a caretaker, such as an addict like Mom or Dad. They become free to choose, which is the goal of helping families escape from their roles that support the addict.

SCAPEGOAT/DISTRACTOR

The family hero is a tough act to follow. In fact, most would believe that it is impossible to compete with his or her achievements and accomplishments. Rather than try, the distractor of the family takes a different course, a course that diverts attention away from the main source of conflict and pain, the addict. The scapegoat becomes the problem child. All energy is channeled into negative and destructive behaviors. At a quick glance, one would think it is a form of modeling after the addict's role. But it is more than that; it is a way to seek recognition and attention in a family whose members are rigidly restrained from reaching out to each other.

The scapegoat goes beyond the family for a sense of belonging. There are usually strong attachments to peer groups or gangs that are very negative in their reinforcements. The scapegoat, openly hostile, defiant and angry, acts out these negative feelings in antisocial behavior. Talk, dress, and actions are all red flags of rebellion, symbols of the internal conflict of survival. But on the inside, what he or she feels most deeply is guilt. The scapegoat feels guilty about his or her own life and about the life of the addict. The individual feels guilty because of his or her inability to change the family and inability or unwillingness to change himself or herself.

The classic, stereotypical female scapegoat becomes pregnant as a teenager. She begins a new life for herself, or at least attempts to, in a most harmful manner. She escapes from one struggling family and starts one of her own. The typical male scapegoat and distractor is a troublemaker at school from the early days in the classroom. Often this is the family member who also becomes an addict. Later, the individual has great difficulty holding down a steady job. Often the end result of the antisocial role is a lifetime in prison. This distractor certainly achieves the goal of taking the focus off the alcoholic or addict, but in so doing, he causes yet another life to be wasted by addiction.

When change occurs in the life of the scapegoat, it appears to be more profound than in the other roles. Because of their ability to live on the visceral edge of reality, recovering scapegoats can see and accept total reality better than most. They become very courageous individuals who put back into this world far more than they receive. They contribute to the well-being of others, learn to accept responsibility, and live productive lives. People often turn to them for help. They make excellent counselors, therapists, and consultants. The sadness of their early years is often turned into happiness and meaning, which they spread to others around them.

QUIET/LOST CHILD

Quiet/lost children never get too close to anyone. They become the forgotten child of their families. Providing a sense of relief because they are never a problem, quiet/lost children stick to themselves and carry on with life without a whimper. People take notice and comment on how well-mannered and nice they are, but that is about the only comment they get. They are almost invisible in their existence. They are not troublemakers, but without help, these withdrawn loners are in deep trouble.

Quiet/lost children have very few friends. They pick up a friend for a while only to follow and watch. There is little if any indication of a relationship. They attach themselves to things, not people. Things have less potential to hurt than people, so they attempt to find comfort in them.

The needs of these lost children go unnoticed for most of their lives. In their withdrawn and detached state, they certainly do not express their needs to anyone. They appear completely self-sufficient to anyone who comes close. But on the inside, they experience deep loneliness and need. They long to be close but are stuck in a role that will not allow intimacy. They live by the motto: "If you don't get too close, you won't get hurt." In living with a family that has constant pain, they set out to avoid pain at all costs.

The lost or quiet children in addicted families are often the future depressives of our society. They have little energy or zest for living. Later they may take one of two distinctly different paths. One path will take them into extreme promiscuity. On this path they attach themselves to another person emotionally for a short while only and move on to another before they get too close to get hurt. The other course is one of complete loneliness and isolation for an entire lifetime. Frequently, the struggle between these two routes results in sexual identity problems. Internal conflict manifests itself in many forms of early death for these sad strugglers.

With help, these lonely and lifeless ones can become some of the most self-actualized people around. They have searched the depths of their souls and found emptiness within. Once they begin to recover, they extend themselves to be a part of life. They grab for and do those things that provide the most meaning. They are creative people, who can produce art and literature from their imagination and talents. They can become the people who are most envied because of their unique ability to design a world of beauty around themselves. When in recovery, their words are few, but when they speak, people listen for meaning and depth. Because of this, it is sad to see so few lost children break out of their roles. When they refuse to, we all miss out on the quality that they can add to life.

MASCOT/COMEDIAN

The mascot or comedian in the family of the addict learns to cope in a completely different way than others do. These personalities immaturely learn to laugh away every painful event; they certainly try to, anyway. Their humor and laughter are inappropriate, given the severity of the situation. But it is their way both to divert attention away from the addict and attract attention for themselves. They find that humor can momentarily soothe the family pain, and it can put them in the spotlight for a while. But it clashes with the frustration and sorrow of the other family members.

On the outside, you would observe fun and humor, the ability always to have a very good time. Nothing in life is too serious to destroy a smile. This is only a protective outer shell hiding a very fragile and afraid individual. They fear the ultimate destruction of the addict, the family, and themselves. They fear the day when their inadequacy to cope is "found out."

Without help, the comedians of the family frequently remain immature for a lifetime. They move from class clown to neighborhood prankster to company joker. These people who feel so unloved and unimportant never learn the complete array of social skills. They stick to their old ways of diversion and denial of problems. Unaided, they remain hyperactive and with short attention spans. Many suffer from learning disabilities. Their inability to cope with stress in a mature, productive manner often results in ulcers and other stress-related diseases. Their inadequacy often leads them into a relationship with a former family hero, someone who can take care of all the problems too cumbersome to bear.

With help, the clowns of the family become most enjoyable people to be with. They develop a good sense of humor and can be favorites in a crowd of friends once recovery brings balance to life. Though immature from years of inadequacy, they grow up fast and mature into wonderful people. They no longer have to laugh to fight back the tears.

It does not matter what adversity comes our way in life. What matters is how we react and what we do with the adversity. This is especially true for every member of the codependent family. Each person struggles to survive. That struggle can trap them in an optionless role of few behaviors or choices, but it does allow them to survive. And the survival process can add strength where there is weakness in others. On that strength can be built a life full of character, meaning, purpose, and true, wonderful love.

It is not easy to break out of a role that has been a habit for years. It is hard to face the pain of change and the challenge of learning a new way to live. But it is never too late. Anyone can reach down with all his or her might and strength, as little as it may seem, and spring from the family trap of addiction. Anyone can break free into a world of relationships full of choices and options. It is not necessary to play out a predictable role that ends in misery and dissatisfaction. One can develop one's own role, composed of nothing but oneself, meaningful relationships, God, and well-deserved love. The struggle of life exists within every man, woman, and child. The beauty in life comes when that struggle is to find a better way. The ugly part of life comes from struggling to stay the same. No matter what stage of the struggle, anyone can change. Anyone can turn his or her struggle into a means of finding a new life far beyond the sick roles of a sick family. Recovery is available to all. When a co-dependent family enters recovery, freedom results for every member.

CHAPTER SEVEN

THE PROGRESSION

Alcoholism is a mystery to most people. They have no idea how it starts or how it develops. In fact, though, it follows a very predictable progression. Myth and misinformation have produced a tainted view of how alcoholism starts and progresses. Most people view the progression as composed of these stages:

1. THE ABSTAINER.   This is the stage at which a person has not yet consumed any alcohol. For some, this stage ends very early in life. Others spend their whole lives as abstainers. But most people, by the time they have completed high school, have progressed to the next stage.

2. THE EXPERIMENTER.   It is at this stage that a person experiences alcohol for the first time. It extends through the time that a person has tried straight whiskey, beer, and two or three different types of wine. For some, these first drinking experiences are pleasurable, but for many, alcohol is merely consumed because it is a sign of maturity and acceptance in society. After the experimentation phase, some return to abstention and remain there for a lifetime, but most progress to the next stage.

3. THE SOCIAL DRINKER.   It is in this stage that most people end up and stay for the rest of their lives. Most believe that people who drink socially do so only because they want to be social. There is a popular claim that social drinkers, unlike alcoholics, do not drink to feel the effect of alcohol, that a social drinker would not use the alcohol as a means of relaxing or coping with a very difficult day. In addition, the social drinker is supposedly in control of the drinking at all times. If he or she does not stick to the social standards of acceptable drinking behavior, then the move into the next stage toward alcoholism occurs.

4. THE IRRESPONSIBLE DRINKER.   This stage characterizes the person who does not simply drink to be sociable.

Society holds that the person who drinks alone on occasion is drinking irresponsibly and is in danger of crossing an imaginary line and reaching to the final stage of alcoholism. Irresponsible drinking is also identified in the person who becomes intoxicated repeatedly. This often leads to a drunk-driving conviction, which is outright proof of irresponsible drinking.

5. THE ALCOHOLIC.   Society says that this stage is the result of not coping with life; the person who reaches this stage has been irresponsible in many areas of life, and, as a just reward, the person becomes an alcoholic. In this view, one year a person could be a normal drinker and the next year have crossed over the line into alcoholism. The alcoholic has been an irresponsible drinker, and the way to prevent alcoholism is to teach people to drink responsibly.

It sounds very logical, doesn't it? But the facts are quite different. The concept of the imaginary line between irresponsible drinking and alcoholism has a major erroneous component known as self-infliction. Society has determined that alcoholics are the victims of their own choices and that the only way to recover from the problem is for them to realize what they have done to themselves. This view of alcoholism is not only false but very destructive. It has prevented many people from receiving the treatment they needed and deserved.

The evidence shows that alcoholism is not a self-inflicted malady but a disease caused by a genetic predisposition. It is a disease not because the alcoholic ends up with a diseased body, like cirrhosis of the liver, but because it is in and of itself an abnormal physical condition. You will often hear professionals speak of the disease concept of alcoholism where they are actually referring to a mental or psychological disease concept of the problem. Alcoholism is not a mental illness or a psychological disorder; it is a primary *physiological* illness that produces drastic psychological, social, and spiritual consequences. This is such a difficult idea for many to accept that changes in attitude are slow in coming. But the evidence of millions of alcoholic lives is overwhelming. To see the evidence, one must be willing to move beyond biases that are supported by myth, not fact.

Facts support the view that a mental disorder does not form the basis for alcoholism. A person with a mental disorder can also be alcoholic, but most alcoholics do not have extraordinary

Society's view of the progression:

IMAGINARY LINE

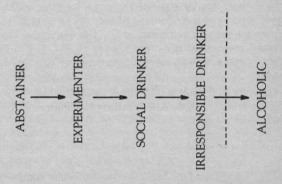

ABSTAINER → EXPERIMENTER → SOCIAL DRINKER → IRRESPONSIBLE DRINKER → ALCOHOLIC

mental problems that produce alcoholism. The history of most alcoholics reveals that their psychological distress was no greater than others' *when* the drinking began, but as the alcoholism progressed, psychological as well as social and spiritual problems intensified. Studies of recovering alcoholics have shown that in only about 5 percent of the cases was there a preexisting mental disorder. For the majority, treatment for the disease of alcoholism is all that is needed to restore a person to a normal life.

The alcoholic is someone who is a victim of a disease that is genetic and developmental in nature. There is a genetic predisposition that develops over time, if accompanied by drinking. A person born with a genetic predisposition to alcoholism and raised in a heavy-drinking environment where there is continued exposure to alcohol will be highly susceptible to the disease. When alcohol enters a body that is biologically susceptible to the problem, the progression of alcoholism begins. If the person is not susceptible to alcoholism, only two alternatives exist: normal drinking or problem drinking. The characteristics of these two practices are very different from the alcoholism progression.

Two important factors of alcoholic progression are consistently shown in the lives of alcoholics. One is that the progression is irreversible; once it begins, it cannot be arrested. Over and over, those who have stopped drinking for years and then relapsed report that their drinking problem picks up as if there had been no years of abstinence at all. The destructive clock cannot be reversed once the progression begins, and in fact appears to speed up with every futile attempt to stop the progression.

The second important point about the progression is that it is terminal. If the alcoholic does not receive treatment of some type or ultimately go insane, the progression ends in death. That death usually does not come as a result of a diseased liver or some other organ damaged by vast quantities of alcohol. Instead, the death of the alcoholic is caused most often by an automobile accident or fire or drowning or some other catastrophe resulting from the drinking, while the alcoholic's organs are still healthy.

The progression of alcoholism begins when the first drink is consumed. With that first drink something different happens in the body of the alcoholic that does not occur in the body of the normal drinker. In the body of the normal drinker there is a predictable reaction to the alcohol. That reaction is the effect that the alcohol produces. It is this effect that has caused human beings to produce alcoholic beverages in various forms for thousands of years. The effect is different in form for each individual and depends a lot on a person's expectation of the alcohol. For some the effect is relaxation; for others it is a lift or a boost of energy; for most there is some type of euphoria. This effect is the reason people drink. People do not drink to be social or because wine goes well with meals; they drink because of the way alcohol can make them feel. The social drinker is no different from the alcoholic in why he or she drinks. They both drink because of the way alcohol makes people feel. The difference is in what happens once that drink is ingested.

Unlike that of the social drinker, the system of the alcoholic does not react predictably to the alcohol. When alcohol enters a biologically susceptible body, what is known as adaptation develops. In this process of adaptation, the system of the alcoholic begins to adapt to the alcohol on the cellular level. Laboratory studies support these findings. Research done at the University of California, San Francisco, has found signs of a genetic difference in cells that could help identify people likely to become alcoholics. Cells from alcoholics appear to be biochemically different and adapt more quickly to alcohol than do cells taken from a nonalcoholic.*

When alcohol enters the system, it changes enzymes, hormones, and numerous chemical processes. In an effort to counteract these changes, the cells alter their structure and method of function. Eventually the cells begin to work smoothly and efficiently with alcohol in the system as the adaptation process continues. The end result of the adaptation is a cell structure that will choose alcohol over other substances and food sources, producing a craving for the chemical when it is absent from the body.

In the alcoholic, the drinking changes the system into one that functions well on alcohol. The individual in the early stages of alcoholism will report that alcohol is not a problem at all, and that, in fact, when the person is drinking, he or she feels more normal than when not drinking. This is not a sign of weakness or the need to escape; it is a symptom of a body that has become accustomed to processing alcohol. The system prefers to function with alcohol in it, and this leads to more and more drinking. The heavy drinking is a result of the system's adaptation to the alcohol; the adaptation is not a result of heavy drinking. The heavy drinking could not have occurred unless the adaptation process had begun.

When the adaptation begins, two things occur within the body of the drinker. One is that the system in effect begs for more and more of the chemical. This is often mistaken for a compulsion to drink. It is not a compulsion from the mind, it is a form of craving from the body. The second thing that happens in the adaptation process is that more and more of the chemical is needed to produce the same effect. So the alcoholic, continuing to drink for the same reason as everyone else, has two complicating factors involved with the drinking process. The body has adapted to the chemical and prefers to function with it in the

*"Study Finds Difference in Cells Of Alcoholics," New York Times, (Thursday, September, 14, 1988) 23.

system, and more and more of the alcohol is required. If this adaptation did not occur, the progression of alcoholism would not continue.

When a normal drinker consumes too much, a limiting mechanism within him or her automatically prevents tolerance from increasing. That automatic limiting mechanism has several forms: Some people fall asleep after only a small amount of alcohol; others become very ill after only a couple of drinks (this reaction can be intensified due to inherited metabolism of certain races); still others become so drunk on a little alcohol that consumption is automatically cut off. These limiting mechanisms prevent the tolerance of a social drinker from climbing precipitously like that of the alcoholic. It is the major indicator distinguishing alcoholism from social drinking.

If you plotted the tolerance of a social drinker over a lifetime, it would look something like this:

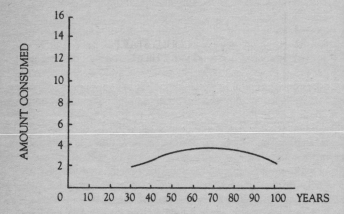

The tolerance of the social drinker may fluctuate from time to time because of illness or the amount of food consumed before drinking, but overall it remains basically level throughout his or her lifetime. It gradually increases with age and then gradually tapers off. With the social drinker, it takes only a few drinks to produce the predictable effect of euphoria or relaxation. Any more than that has a different effect entirely, and that predictable negative effect automatically limits how much alcohol can be drunk. With the alcoholic, that is not so.

The increasing tolerance for alcohol is the first observable indication of alcoholism. As the adaptation process continues, the alcoholic, lacking the limiting mechanisms that characterize the social drinker, can consume a volume of alcohol that amazes all who look on. The social drinker will become very ill, fall asleep, or get too drunk to consume any more alcohol when the drinking is excessive, but the alcoholic will not. As a result, the alcoholic's tolerance is able to continue to rise.

The tolerance pattern of the alcoholic is a predictable one. It usually begins low, increases to an extremely high level, and eventually, in the later stages, it drops off significantly. Plotting the tolerance for the alcoholic gives us something like this:

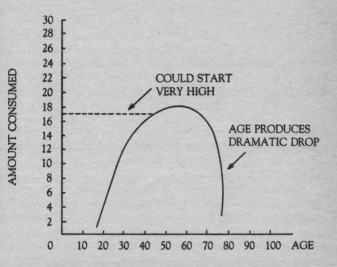

One difference that some alcoholics may experience is a very high initial tolerance, but for most it begins at a normal low level. At the point at which tolerance begins to rise, alcoholism and its progression are well under way. The observable problems do not occur until later, after the tolerance is high, but the progression begins long before the development of problems. Prevention programs will be most effective when they attempt to stop the drinking problem in the early stages. It is not necessary to wait until a life is almost over or completely destroyed before detecting the presence of alcoholism.

Once the tolerance remains high, the alcoholic will begin to realize that the body actually improves its performance as the drinking continues throughout the day. If a social drinker were to begin drinking at five o'clock and continue to drink throughout the evening, the normal result would be some degree of impaired performance. The signs of drunkenness would eventually reveal that the social drinker has consumed beyond the level of his or her tolerance. For the alcoholic, whose tolerance is high, the first drink of the evening would begin a process of feeling more and more normal. Performance will not be affected until the alcoholic drinks beyond his or her tolerance, and for many alcoholics, this rarely occurs. It is not unusual to know of someone who rarely becomes drunk, never causes any problems in the family, but just seems always to have a drink in one hand. This person is in total control of his or her drinking and certainly would not drink at unacceptable times, such as during work hours. But what is present is the beginning of a progression that will cause tremendous problems in life. This early stage, although invisible to most people, indicates that drinking for the alcoholic is not the same as for other social drinkers. There are many people still in this stage whose drinking is not normal, and their defensiveness about their drinking has already begun. They proclaim their ability to control their drinking and to stop at any time. The fact that control is an issue at all is a strong indicator of alcoholism.

One of the baffling aspects of the disease of alcoholism is that the timing differs for each individual. Some alcoholics continue maintenance drinking for many years; what they would call normal social drinking is actually controlled alcoholic drinking. For others with the predisposition to alcoholism, the ability to control the drinking is very short-lived. Whether there is one year or twenty years of controlled drinking, when the tolerance is high, it is alcoholism, whether the person is in control or not. Alcoholism does not mysteriously develop when the control is lost; it is present, and progressing, on every occasion when the alcoholic drinks twice as much as someone else, or whenever everyone is drunk on a little alcohol and the person is not affected after a great quantity.

Throughout the early stages of alcoholism, the addiction pro-

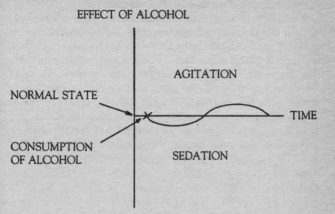

cess increases its influence on the life of the alcoholic. The adaptation leads to more and more drinking because the body actually craves the chemical. But the addiction process is also intensified by the production of the highly addictive THIQ substance. As was presented in Chapter four, the social drinker does not produce this chemical. When normal drinkers have consumed one drink, they have advanced the addiction process one drink's worth, but for the alcoholic, that one drink produces a greater amount of addiction because of the production of THIQ. This is another physiological process unique to the alcoholic that complicates the drinking and drives him or her deeper into the addiction.

The next factor in the progression is the withdrawal effect. Tolerance is a key element here because a person must be able to consume a lot of alcohol for withdrawal to be a problem. Most people are aware that alcohol is an addictive chemical. The more a person drinks, the deeper he or she goes into the addiction process. If someone were to become ill on only two drinks, he or she would never experience the results of the withdrawal process. When a person consumes one can of beer, there will be one can of beer's worth of withdrawal—that is, a sensation of agitation following the initial sedation. But since one can of beer contains so little alcohol, the drinker would not be aware of that withdrawal taking place. The graph above plots the sedative effect of that beer and the agitation level of withdrawal compared to a normal mood level. The difference is very small.

For the alcoholic able to consume vast quantities of alcohol, it is a different matter. Three six-packs' worth of withdrawal or three bottles of wine's worth of withdrawal or a bottle of vodka's worth of withdrawal are much different from one beer's worth of withdrawal. The alcoholic's withdrawal will radically affect the way in which the person functions and relates to other people after the drinking has stopped. Plotting the alcoholic's drinking, sedation, and agitation makes it obvious that the withdrawal from large quantities of alcohol produces an affected person, a person who is not the same as before the drinking began. (Remember, because of a unique process of metabolism, the alcoholic will not experience as much sedation from one drink as a social drinker. This is due to the increase in tolerance. Note also that the alcoholic experiences the agitating effect of withdrawal immediately after he or she experiences the sedative effects of the currently consumed drink, a highly stressful conflict.)

Consider the young executive whose tolerance has gone up and who is in the initial stages of alcoholism. He leaves work at five-thirty to have a drink with his associates, but the associates have a drink and the executive has two doubles. By seven, the man is at home having a couple of beers before dinner. At dinner he splits a bottle of wine with his wife. She has one glass and he has the remainder of the bottle. After dinner he has a drink while finishing up some paperwork and then goes to bed. In four and a half hours, he consumes the equivalent of eleven drinks with little or no noticeable effect.

To many, this is an example of a normal social drinker who is in control of his drinking. He's not drinking at work, driving while intoxicated, or abusing his wife. In reality, this is the classic picture of the alcoholic in the early stages. The result of taking in this much alcohol during a normal evening may not seem too great, but it is a fairly large dose of an addictive chemical. When morning comes, the executive will be experiencing some mild withdrawal symptoms, such as slight agitation and moodiness. He will think he is normal, that his personality has merely developed a low frustration tolerance. He will not associate his mood of the morning with the drinking of the previous evening.

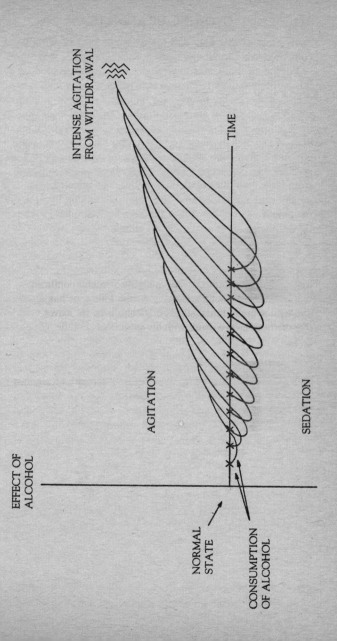

And what about the times that the young executive overdoes it? On a Friday evening after a tough week, after-work drinks may double and carry over into a social event where heavy drinking goes on well into the night. Saturday morning, one of the few times he spends with his children, will be noticeably affected by the previous night's drinking. The increased agitation and moodiness will progress to some more devastating symptoms for the alcoholic and his family. What the alcoholic may call a hangover is actually withdrawal. He may experience any of the symptoms characteristic of the withdrawal syndrome:

Shakiness	Nausea
Insomnia	Increased perspiration
Headache	Moodiness
Eye ache	Depression

Any of these, in isolation or in combination with other symptoms, is enough to change the executive's interaction with his children on Saturday morning. When the kids are not perfect, make too much noise and disturb Dad's sleep, he may awaken angry and obsessed with his own discomfort—a condition hardly conducive to spending quality time with the family.

One symptom of withdrawal is guaranteed to continue to progress: the growing desire to remedy the other symptoms. This may be under control for years before it presents an obvious problem, but the alcoholic will increasingly become aware that when he drinks, he feels more "normal" than when he is not drinking. Because alcohol temporarily relieves the symptoms of addiction, the alcoholic feels more at ease, both physically and mentally. His family may even encourage drinking, knowing the alcoholic is easier to manage with a drink than without. (Of course, this applies to the "dry" alcoholic and not the "recovering" alcoholic.) Later the family may feel that their encouragement for the alcoholic to drink caused the alcoholism, and this increases their guilt.

The young executive will continue to drink in control, at times in moderation, at others to excess. Withdrawal symptoms will become more intense, and the need to drink to relieve them will increase. The executive may find himself in the category of a maintenance drinker. Maintenance drinkers rarely get intoxicated but are frequently drinking to maintain a feeling of normality and to ward off the withdrawal symptoms. Maintenance drinkers have a tolerance so high that rarely do they drink beyond it. Above their tolerance, maintenance drinkers are intoxicated and out of control, but below it, they just seem to drink a lot. Either way, they are continuing to saturate themselves with an addictive chemical and then withdrawing from the chemical. Again, this produces a person who is not normal. The personality changes as the addiction process increases its grip on every aspect of the alcoholic's life. If the alcoholic had not been able to drink a lot of alcohol, if the person's tolerance had not been tremendously high, the addiction process and the resulting withdrawal syndrome would have never occurred.

As the problem progresses, the withdrawal syndrome also progresses. Undetectable at first, it becomes more severe, reaching a point of almost unbearable agitation. Eventually withdrawal presents a far greater problem than mere increased agitation. It can become a hellish nightmare of hallucinations, convulsions, and delirium tremens; crawling bugs, snakes, demons, and monsters often attack the advanced alcoholic's mind while in withdrawal. Withdrawal may one day kill the alcoholic, but more likely, death will result from some other consequence of the alcoholism, such as a traffic accident.

Another result of the alcoholic's ability to drink vast quantities of alcohol is toxicity, which occurs when one drinks more alcohol than the liver can detoxify. Toxicity is not to be confused with intoxication, the loss of control of behavior from drinking over one's tolerance. Toxicity is an entirely different phenomenon, observable when the alcoholic is not intoxicated. Someone who is toxic may not have had a drink for days. During the detoxification phase of treatment, intoxication is over within hours, but toxicity will last for days. Toxicity damages a person's will and ability to think, feel, remember, and judge. The entire personality is distorted by toxins that hamper the functioning of the central nervous system.

The amount of alcohol consumed determines whether it should be classified as a food, drug, or poison. In the beginning, the alcoholic drinks alcohol in amounts so small that it could be considered a food substance, since it provides calories to the body. As drinking continues and mood is affected, it could be considered a socially acceptable mood-altering drug. But the alcoholic consumes it in such large quantities that it becomes a deadly poison, destroying the mind and body and undermining the health of the drinker. The alcoholic's body is unable to rid itself of the toxic chemicals found in the alcohol.

Because the alcoholic drinks enough alcohol for it to be considered a poison, the brain is adversely affected. What the brain is supposed to do, it does in a sick way. As the ability to detoxify the body lessens, more and more toxins remain in the system and collect in the brain. The greater the amount consumed, the greater the toxicity. The more toxic a person becomes, the less rationally he or she is able to think, yet often those around the toxic alcoholic are expecting an irrational, damaged brain to make the rational decision to get well. The distorted brain chemistry prevents normal brain functioning and traps the alcoholic more firmly in the disease. When an alcoholic stops drinking, it can be months or years before the body, mind, and spirit are free from the damage inflicted by the toxins. The psychological economy of the toxic alcoholic is destroyed, and he or she cannot relate normally to others. The distorted personality and the mental and emotional difficulties become too intense to hide.

This stage of alcoholism is the one most frequently identified. Fearing a breakdown or collapse, the alcoholic finally reaches out for some sort of help. Once the psychological problems are severe enough, the alcoholic usually talks to a professional counselor, minister, or physician about the drinking. When he or she discusses the problems and the amount of drinking, the professional consulted may assume that the drinking is a way to cope with all the psychological problems, but these did not erupt until the drinking increased to such high levels. The drinking is not a consequence of the psychological problems; the psychological problems are a consequence of the drinking. Attempting to resolve psychological turmoil and conflict will not eliminate the drinking problem, which must be dealt with directly rather than as a symptom of a greater underlying problem.

For the alcoholic, life becomes increasingly more miserable as the drinking continues to impair the mind. The toxins prevent thinking and memory from functioning naturally. *Emotional augmentation* best describes the state of feelings: the feelings of the alcoholic become more extreme; bad moods become deep depressions, and agitation becomes intense anger. Discussions end in argument, and arguments often end in physical abuse. The alcoholic is out of control emotionally and has lost the ability to control his or her behavior. Until the body is fully detoxified and free of the toxins, the mind will function abnormally.

The toxic alcoholic has difficulty in concentrating. Obsession with discomfort and the need to relieve the withdrawal symptoms are enough to impair concentration; add brain toxicity, and the alcoholic has little chance of functioning with a sharp mind. Decisions are difficult to make and are quite often inconsistent and inappropriate. The thinking process of even the most brilliant minds decays as the alcoholism continues to progress.

In addition to these mental and psychological problems, the alcoholic experiences memory loss. He or she may forget meetings, dates, agreements, and entire evenings as the toxins from the alcohol interfere with the brain's nerve impulses. Blackouts will occur in which the alcoholic appears to be functioning normally but will not be able to remember anything that happened. People have come out of a blackout and found themselves on an airplane, not knowing how they boarded the plane or where it was going. This frightening experience can motivate recovery. Memory is a vital tool for life, and when it becomes unreliable, the alcoholic, deep inside, becomes very frightened. Rarely will the alcoholic know that the source of the problem is drinking. More than likely the self-diagnosis will be "I must be losing my mind."

These problems combine to produce self-doubt, fear, and a very unstable person. The instability increases as the progression of alcoholism continues. The alcoholic knows that something must be done to prevent losing all control; some try intense exercise, some turn to psychoanalysis—anything just to hang on. He or she will attempt many different things in an effort to retain stability, but any positive result will be temporary at best. The alcoholic may resort to total abstinence, but stopping drinking without starting recovery only makes the problems worse and the psychological pain greater. The progression keeps the alcoholic from having any idea what will happen, but he or she does know things are not getting better. Somewhere along the way the old self has vanished. Days of depressed inactivity followed by days of impulsive decisions and actions confuse the alcoholic and those close to the alcoholic. To the alcoholic, life is now a painful and hopeless exercise in futility.

As the disease progresses, everyone close to the alcoholic will be affected adversely. This is most noticeable in the alcoholic's intimate relationships. If the alcoholic is full of fear, self-doubt, and emptiness, he or she cannot develop or maintain a solid relationship with a husband, wife, girlfriend or boyfriend. The alcoholic knows the problem is much worse but does not know the others are aware of that. Lying and deception are used to cover up the severity of the problem. The need to deny its severity will build a wall of distrust that grows higher and wider with each new discussion of the drinking. Eventually a marriage under these circumstances will no longer be a marriage but continue as a sick arrangement where both people lose their desire to be married. They stay together for the kids, appearances, or some other reason than that of two people striving to meet each other's needs.

The alcoholic's children will also suffer the consequences of the drinking. Their confusion over the love they feel and the behavior they see will distort their concept of adult roles and relationships. The alcoholic will guiltily try to be the perfect parent. When the drinking episodes explode into family disaster, the alcoholic will recoil with attempts to regain control, which become more and more futile as time passes. Like the spouse, the children will begin to experience the wall of distrust; they will find themselves in a double bind of not trusting the parent but having no alternative except to trust.

The relationship between the alcoholic and the children has no chance of normality. Even when drinking episodes stop, the brain is affected by the toxic chemicals and the central nervous system is in a constant state of adjustment. Every interaction has a foundation of memories of strange behavior and fear of what is going to happen next. The children begin to isolate and move away from the alcoholic. First they move out emotionally, then they leave physically. It is done not to hurt, but to survive.

The children of the alcoholic will suffer some traumatic, life-changing experiences. Physical and verbal abuse and incest will permanently scar the children, the relationships, and the family. The alcoholic's guilt and remorse and the compensation for the negative actions and feelings will only lead to greater, and disastrous, attempts at control. Everyone involved needs intensive therapy for recovery from these devastating events. Until therapy begins, survival is about all the children can hope for.

The nondrinker or nonalcoholic has a very difficult time understanding how alcoholism can lead a person toward violence and perversion. Even an alcoholic who is still in control, continuing to nurture his or her children, finds it hard to relate to the alcoholic who has been involved in physical abuse or incest. The power and force of the disease are beyond most people's comprehension. Often the progression leads the healthiest of parents to act so destructive as to destroy any hope for a normal life for the kids. This is probably the worst consequence of the progression: children damaged for life because of the ignorance surrounding the alcoholic and alcoholism. As the children fight to survive, they miss many aspects of normal development. There is rarely, if ever, any happiness for them. In later life, the sad situation of their own childhood is often repeated and played out in the families they produce—sickness begets sickness.

The problems go far beyond the family, into every part of the alcoholic's life. No area is immune from alcoholism's effects. Sooner or later, work performance will be affected and the job will be jeopardized; the alcoholic's productivity is weakened by the bodily toll the disease takes. By the time this happens, the disease will have progressed into the middle and later stages. The family problems will very likely have resulted in divorce and behavior problems with the children; those children able to do so may have already abandoned the family. It is common for alcoholics to lose their families but do anything possible to save their jobs.

Often job performance actually improves early in this stage of the progression. When the alcoholic loses control at home and senses problems developing in other areas, he or she will compensate by working extra hard to prove that "I've got it" or "I'm still in control." But because of how alcoholism destroys the psychological economy, it is not long before the employer and fellow employees know that the man or woman who was hired is not the same man or woman there now. Eventually the alcoholic will be in a career crisis because of the drinking.

The problems with the job will inevitably have a financial impact on the alcoholic's life. Promotions will be missed, performance bonuses not earned, and pay cuts even may ensue. Other financial difficulties will occur. Drinking up the paycheck or just spending a large percentage of the salary on alcohol will cause problems; potential investments will be missed because of money wasted on booze; and because of the malfunctioning brain, irrational and inappropriate financial decisions will be made. The tendency to overspend is very common. A typical example is the alcoholic who gets drunk, then takes his wife on a trip they both know they cannot afford but she feels she deserves. It is his inappropriate way to prove he can be wonderful. Both spouses get seduced into this pattern of repeated pain and reward. The pain is increased when the bills come in to finance the inappropriate rewards.

For most alcoholics, the financial strains become greater as the disease progresses. Financial crises often precipitate the quest for treatment. But for some, finances are never a problem. They have almost unlimited resources, and for them, financial problems mean opportunities lost or money not made. Whatever the situation, if someone does not intervene, the alcoholic will have to deal with what drinking has done to the financial potential. Early intervention can save thousands of dollars for the alcoholic and the alcoholic's family.

Legal problems may also develop. Driving while intoxicated or drunk and disorderly behavior will land many alcoholics in jail. Many attorneys are skilled in getting the alcoholic off alcohol-related charges, but this only allows the alcoholic to continue to drink without experiencing the immediate consequences. Getting the alcoholic off on a drunk-driving charge is a terrible way to make a living; it kills people. There is always also the possibility of something happening that is not so easily handled by an attorney or resolved by paying a fine.

One evening, a member of Alcoholics Anonymous went to a prison to conduct an AA meeting for the prisoners. While he was there, he met a man who was serving a sentence for manslaughter and heard his story. The prisoner had drunk for years, never knowing how serious his problem was. One morning after a night of heavy drinking, he was awakened by his wife's screams from the garage. He shuffled out of bed and into the garage to see the source of her horror. The night before, he had been in a blackout. He could remember nothing about where he had been or how he drove to his house. But on the way home, he had hit a small child with his van. The wife was screaming because the child's body was still attached to the bumper of the van. He was found guilty of manslaughter and sentenced to twenty-five years in prison. A tragic story, but it has been and will be repeated many times over in the lives of other alcoholics. Tragedy is alcoholism's most common symptom. The only unusual aspect of this one is the severity of the sentence; it is disgracefully common for such cases to result in a short prison term or none at all.

Physiological deterioration is the last stage in alcoholic progression. The body is not meant to exist saturated with an addictive chemical that is toxic and an irritant to the entire system. Studies show that alcoholics die about sixteen years earlier than other people. The alcohol causes deterioration in every area of the body. Most people think of the liver when they think of physical complications from alcohol, but the entire system is impaired. In the later stages, the internal physical problems become so serious that the alcoholic drinks to relieve the aches and pains brought about by a body that is deteriorating rapidly. This last stage in the progression is extremely painful, physically and mentally.

The addiction's grip is quite obvious in this stage. Watching a person suffer from pancreatitis and its severe pain, it is easy to realize that only something as powerful as addiction could get the person to drink again. The mental pain compounds this, since willpower and determination are no match for the power of addiction. The alcoholic's existence in this stage can best be described as "deathly emptiness."

The occasional dramatic news story of a movie star or other celebrity who, toward the end of life, surrounded by walls and bodyguards, hides away and drinks until death occurs is paralleled less spectacularly by the experience of thousands of last-stage alcoholics. What was once a form of survival becomes a tool for suicide as physical and mental pain create a bottomless pit of despair. The hope for the alcoholic is that someone will intervene before the disease progresses to this point. If there were no help or no understanding of the problem, it would be simple to comprehend why alcoholism so often reaches the late stages before it is treated, if it ever is. But help is available almost everywhere. For any alcoholic willing to do whatever it takes, the progression can end today.

THE PROGRESSION IN SUMMARY

Early Stage

During the early stage of alcoholism, the alcoholic appears to be "blessed" with the ability to drink a lot of alcohol. There is nothing noticeably different from others about the alcoholic except for the amount of alcohol consumed. The alcoholic can drink much more than others and experience much less effect. The tolerance either starts high or increases over the individual's drinking history.

There is no pain or illness and no immediate obvious penalties for the drinking. There is no threat to career status, and all relationships appear intact. The alcoholic feels great when drinking and can stop at any time. The alcoholism at this stage is invisible to most and appears to be a problem to no one. From time to time the alcoholic will receive praise for the ability to drink a lot—but what is being praised are the early symptoms of alcoholism.

Middle Stage

In the middle stage of alcoholism, some new reasons for drinking develop. Like everyone else, the alcoholic starts drinking for the effect of the alcohol. Whether it is for a lift or to relax, the initial reason for drinking remains, but more and more these reasons are replaced by drinking to relieve both physical and psychological pain. In this stage, physical dependency and addiction are definitely present. The alcoholic can still maintain periods of abstinence, but it is very difficult, as withdrawal often drives the alcoholic back into drinking.

Craving the chemical is another symptom of the middle stage of alcoholism. The alcoholic begins to expect a drink at a certain time, or associate drinking with many events. When the drink is not available, the alcoholic craves a drink and is obsessed with alcohol. The alcoholic may go days without a drink, but put in a situation where drinking is expected, like a baseball game or a party, he or she will not be able to relax until alcohol is consumed. Because of the grip of addiction, alcohol becomes a major focus in the alcoholic's life. He or she acquires the label of "heavy drinker."

The middle stage is also characterized by problems of control. Sometimes the alcoholic loses control of the drinking. A battle begins to convince everyone that the drinking is manageable. The alcoholic will say things like "I can handle it" or "I'm still in control." The irony is that only an alcoholic would be trying to convince himself or herself and everyone else that he or she is still in control of the drinking. People without a drinking problem do not have to convince anyone of anything about drinking.

The alcoholic loses control in other areas of life. Emotional stability becomes harder to maintain. The alcoholic has difficulty coming out of depression or must struggle to settle down from a hyper state. And of course there is loss of control in areas such as the marriage, family, and the job. During this stage the alcoholic knows that something is badly wrong but battles to try to regain control as it continues to slip away.

Late Stage

During the late stage, all the obvious consequences of alcoholism manifest themselves. The physiological damage affects the heart, liver, gastrointestinal tract, and respiratory system; the body also suffers from malnutrition due to heavy drinking and poor eating habits. The alcoholic is in constant agony from physiological deterioration, mental confusion, and emotional turmoil. The drink that did the damage is now considered by the alcoholic to be the only medicine that can ease the distress of life. The alcoholic is trapped, knowing that the drinking must stop, but unable to stop because of the entire body craving the chemical. When the alcoholic attempts to stop, the ensuing acute withdrawal drives him or her back to drinking. The late stage of alcoholism is a sad state for anyone. The only hope is that someone will intervene who knows what must be done for recovery to occur.

The alcoholic begins drinking for the same reasons as everyone else but diverges onto a path quite dissimilar to social drinking. Because the person is born with a faulty body chemistry or an inability to process alcohol normally, the alcoholism is set in motion. The system adapts to the chemical, and tolerance develops; more and more of the chemical is needed to produce the same effect. As tolerance goes up, the body becomes physiologically dependent. Withdrawal symptoms start when the drinking stops, and, because so much alcohol is consumed, toxicity begins to affect the way the brain functions. The alcoholic's self-concept is destroyed, and the ability to relate to people is damaged. Spiritual growth stops as separation from God becomes a way of life. Other problems in life crop up, causing more emotional stress and discomfort and an increased reason to drink. Finally, the alcoholic continues to drink so much that the body deteriorates more rapidly, and eventually death or insanity occurs due solely to the inability of the alcoholic to stop drinking.

Alcoholics do not cause themselves to become alcoholic. They cannot prevent their bodies from processing the alcohol as they do. The cause is not a weak will, inadequate nurturing, or inability to cope with life. No obsessive-compulsive personality, passive-aggressive behavior pattern, depression, or insecurity is the source, but a system that malfunctions. The problem continues so long because it is misunderstood by family, friends, professionals, and most of society. In the progression, the real person beneath the disease gets lost along the way. Only complete recovery allows that real person, submerged beneath the drinking, to emerge into normality.

Alcohol is a selectively addictive chemical. For most people, alcohol does not present a problem, but for some, it is a deadly poisonous drug. Those who have a system that processes alcohol abnormally will predictably progress through all the stages of alcoholism unless some type of intervention occurs.

It is the beginning, middle, and end that the body of the alcoholic causes the alcoholism. The disease ravages the mind and the emotions, but it is in the physiology, not the psychology, of the person that alcoholism develops. The alcoholic may seek psychiatric help, participate in a behavior modification program, or do any number of things to control the drinking, but eventually must come to know and accept that no amount of therapy for the mind will change the predisposition of the body. The body will be alcoholic forever, and the only thing the alcoholic can do about that is to not drink forever, one day at a time.

CHAPTER EIGHT

PHYSICAL, MENTAL, AND SPIRITUAL ASPECTS OF ALCOHOLISM

The physical aspects of alcoholism are what is inherited. But to fully understand the problem, the psychological reactions and the spiritual interpretations must be studied. Considerable confusion among both professionals and laymen arises from focusing on one aspect over another, resulting in disagreement on how to deal with the problem and how to promote recovery from it. I will delve into that point in the next chapter, but in this one I will examine how these aspects of the progression differ and how they are manifested.

PHYSICAL PROGRESSION

In the previous chapter on the overall course of the alcoholic progression, I have gone into some detail of its physical aspect. In this section, I will focus more fully on it, of necessity going over some ground already covered so that the presentation here will be complete and connected.

As stated in the previous chapters, it all begins with a body predisposed to alcoholism. All of the results of the predisposed system, the toxicity, and the withdrawal can best be described as emotional augmentation. *Emotional augmentation* means that the intensity of the emotions is heightened. The brain is irritated by the toxins, and, as a result, the feeling centers of the brain do not function normally. The effects of the heavy drinking produce an entire central nervous system that is sick, because it is saturated with toxic and irritating chemicals.

Emotional augmentation is considered the first of the observ-

despair
reactions to punish self
worthlessness
insecurity
alienation
remorse
shame
guilt
SPIRITUAL INTERPRETATIONS

anger	infantile behavior
fear	arrested maturity
projection	personality distortion
rationalization	deterioration of self-image
denial	depression

PSYCHOLOGICAL REACTIONS

confused thinking	loss of control	delirium tremens
emotional augmentation	memory defects	increased need for alcohol
	anguish	

PHYSIOLOGICAL SYMPTOMS

able and progressive symptoms of the physiological progression. Even though this system is identifiable and continues to worsen, it is rarely associated with alcoholism. If everyone could understand this one point, it would radically change the concept of alcoholism. The emotional augmentation sets off the entire progression of compensation and other reactions to alcoholism. It is caused by nothing other than the alcoholic's ability to consume a lot of alcohol.

Because the alcoholic now has greater difficulty coping with emotions, anguish begins to surface. As the chemicals continue to irritate the central nervous system and the emotional augmentation increases, the alcoholic becomes obsessed with fear, worry, anxiety, and frustration. The alcoholic fears that he or she may be going crazy. There is worry that perhaps as the difficulties in coping increase, there may come a day when the ability to cope is completely lost. The frustration comes from not being able to identify the source of the problem and not knowing how to improve things.

Anguish is a word much older than the word *anxiety*. It refers to the combination of physical and mental pain. This combination frequently describes exactly what the alcoholic is going through. The physical pain of hangovers and damaged organs coupled with the mental pain of not knowing how to identify the source of the problem makes for a miserable existence. The alcoholic begins to think that perhaps God has singled him or her out for punishment for some past wrongdoing. It is as if a big black cloud of everything negative and unpleasant about life is hovering over the alcoholic.

In the progression, memory also is damaged by the drinking. *Memory defects* come in several forms, one being general forgetfulness. The alcoholic's sharp mind may have launched a successful career that fizzles out because important names, dates, and people are forgotten. The more toxic the brain becomes, the less it is able to function normally.

Another form of memory defect for the alcoholic is called *blackouts*, touched on in the previous chapter. Blackouts are not to be confused with passing out. Passing out happens when a person drinks so much that he or she falls asleep. Blacking out is not characterized by falling asleep. Everyone around the person in a blackout thinks that the alcoholic is aware of what's going on, but the alcoholic in a blackout will not remember anything that happened.

Blackouts can be very detrimental to an alcoholic's career. During a blackout an executive may very successfully conduct a meeting, make major decisions, and develop a powerful plan of action. Then, to the dismay of the alcoholic and those attending the meeting, the alcoholic is unable to remember anything that happened during the meeting. The only explanation is that the alcoholic was in a blackout. The blackout is considered by many as the major red flag indicating the presence of alcoholism.

Confused thinking eventually results from saturation of the body by alcohol. Because of the toxic brain, the alcoholic finds it difficult to concentrate for long periods of time. Some of the sharpest minds have been dulled into ineffectiveness due to toxicity. At times the most opinionated individuals find themselves wavering from side to side on issues that they would have fought for in the past.

Life for the alcoholic with a toxic brain is like living in a fog or a daze. It is a miracle that more catastrophes do not happen due to the impairment of the brain. This phenomenon can result in a total change in personal morality. Alcoholics become involved in activities and relationships that are not only unhealthy but contradict everything the alcoholic has believed in. This has helped to promote the stigma of alcoholism as a result of "immorality." What has happened is not a choice to abandon personal values, but that the ability to uphold those values has been destroyed by the toxic brain. The confusion in thinking, feeling, and personal values harms the alcoholic and those close to him or her. It also becomes another excuse to drink more. To cope with the guilt and the frustration of this type of existence, full of personal and interpersonal conflict, the alcoholic turns to the bottle.

The next symptom is an indication of the growing power of physical addiction as well as of psychological dependency. This symptom is observed as the *increased need for alcohol*. The alcoholic simply won't go where alcohol is not. For most, that begins the process of eliminating such places as churches and PTA meetings. The life of the alcoholic begins to revolve around the chemical, and he or she is never too far from it. Access is safeguarded by putting a cooler in the trunk, a bottle under the seat, and buying unique gadgets like a cane with a hidden flask. The rules of supply and demand control the alcoholic. The body demands the alcohol, and the alcoholic must stay close to it.

At this point the alcoholic is well into the progression of the disease and discovers that the only temporary cure for the symptoms of distress is more alcohol. But the tolerance is so high that the chemical is consumed in amounts great enough to become a poison. The more of the chemical consumed, the more poisonous it becomes to the body, mind, and spirit. The alcoholic feels he or she can in no way exist without the chemical alcohol or some substitute like Valium. In reality, at this point of the progression, it is life-threatening for many alcoholics to attempt to stop drinking without help.

Loss of control is the classic indicator for alcoholism. Before this loss of control occurs, many deny the addiction. Someone may have lost three wives, three jobs, and had three citations for drunk driving and still claim he is not alcoholic, since he can still control the drinking. But in actuality, all alcoholics are on a collision course with the day when they will no longer be able to control the drinking. They are alcoholic before losing control and after losing control. The difference is that after losing control, it is very difficult to deny the alcoholism.

Loss of control is characterized by the inability to predict the drinking behavior once the drinking has begun. It doesn't mean that a person can't stop drinking for two or three weeks. When the drinking does begin, the desired two drinks become the uncontrollable twenty. Many alcoholics will proclaim that they are not alcoholic because they can still go for certain periods of time without drinking. The effort required to maintain these dry spells is proof enough that alcoholism is in full force.

Loss of control also refers to the inability to control emotions. Emotional augmentation eventually becomes emotional crisis. The alcoholic may find himself or herself breaking into tears or uproarious laughter at inappropriate times. Often at this point, the alcoholic is labeled as having a nervous breakdown. However, these symptoms are not the result of shattered nerves but the end result of a long progression. Once they begin, the alcoholic can be considered as in the late stages of the disease.

The last of the physical symptoms is called *d.t.'s*, or *delirium tremens*. The movies have captured well the horror of hallucinations and severe shakes brought about by the acute withdrawal from alcohol. It is important to note that when most people think of alcoholism, they think of people unable to control their drinking, or skid row bums shaking and hallucinating. The picture of a Madison Avenue executive drinking twelve drinks and functioning normally does not bring to mind alcoholism. Alcoholism begins with the increase in tolerance and ends with loss of control and d.t.'s. All the symptoms in between are just signposts along the progression. There is no imaginary line that one crosses over into alcoholism. Instead, there is a predictable progression that drags the alcoholic through hopeless misery.

These physical symptoms are observable and progressive. They become worse as time goes on. Those around the alcoholic see the symptoms and eventually confront the person with the evidence. The alcoholic, with a fixed image of skid row representing all alcoholics, has predictable reactions to the label "alcoholic" or the suggestion of a drinking problem. As the evidence of the alcoholism intensifies, the reactions from the alcoholic become stronger.

In understanding alcoholism, it is vital to remember that the high tolerance led to the emotional augmentation. What is almost invisible in the beginning surfaces more boldly and more frequently as the progression continues. This progression is predictable, as well as the reaction to the evidence of alcoholism. A lot of people do not accept the basis of these physical symptoms because they focus on the why's of drinking. Remember, drinking is behavioral, and the reasons for it *can* be mental or spiritual, but alcoholism is not behavioral. A person can choose to drink, but no one chooses to be alcoholic. When alcoholism becomes obvious, the psychological reactions predictably begin.

PSYCHOLOGICAL REACTIONS

Denial is the reaction most associated with alcoholism. People are always saying that the worst thing about alcoholics is their extreme denial. If there is one thing that all alcoholics have in common, it is that they deny any problem exists for a long time. Actually, the denial is one of the best things about the alcoholic. It indicates that there remain with the self-contempt some feelings of worth. It is also an indication that the alcoholic does not know what an alcoholic is. When confronted with the evidence of the disease, the alcoholic denies it because he or she thinks that alcoholism is a sign of weakness. Wanting to preserve a sense of strength, the denial is locked in. Or the person may view alcoholics as immoral and need to deny to preserve a sense of goodness. One of the best ways to break through the denial is for the alcoholic to meet other alcoholics who look, talk, act, and drink just like he or she does. That is a key element in the effectiveness of Alcoholics Anonymous and other sources of treatment.

If the brain were not toxic, there would be a much greater chance of the person being persuaded by the obvious consequences of the progression. But the toxicity just reinforces the denial. It produces irrational thoughts and prevents rational decisions. Society's concept of alcoholism also feeds into the denial. The societal view would support denial with such comments as: "Well, he's not on skid row," "He doesn't get drunk any more than anyone else," or "He can stop any time."

Of course, these rationales have nothing to do with whether or not alcoholism exists, but because so many view alcoholism from society's outdated and inaccurate perspective, the denial is reinforced. But when the evidence becomes so strong that complete denial of the problem is impossible, the alcoholic must resort to another tactic of self-destructive "self-preservation." When denial no longer works, rationalization is the next reaction to fall in place.

Rationalization is another form of denial, but with an added dimension. It is an indication that the person recognizes some type of problem exists. In denial, the alcoholic emphatically states that there is no problem. As rationalization develops, there begins to be an admission that there may be a problem of some sort. The rationalizing person says, "I may drink too much on some occasions, but with this high-pressure job, I need to drink. When the job lets up a little, I'll stop drinking or cut back." The alcoholic uses many excuses to make sense of something that doesn't make any sense at all unless the diagnosis of alcoholism is accepted. The alcoholic becomes relentless in the process of rationalization. The family must remember that all rationalizations are attempts to explain the drinking and deny alcoholism. It is admission of a problem so that the focus will be taken off the real problem. The stigma of alcoholism is the reason for so much effort being placed on denial and rationalization. When denial and rationalization prove ineffective, projection is the natural reaction.

The alcoholic retreats back into a stance of total denial and, to secure the position, points to the problems of those close by. This method of denial is called *projection*. If the wife confronts him about his drinking, he will perhaps point to her problem with eating, spending, or working as the actual source of the difficulty. He is likely to tell her that if she would eat less, spend less, or work less, their marriage would be fine. Of course, alcoholics are often very convincing, and the wife is likely to accept some responsibility for the drinking problem. If unaware of this dynamic, the family will be damaged by the alcoholic's indictments. Projection is a destructive reaction and burdens others with guilt and resentment.

Eventually the repeated confrontations begin to wear through the defenses of denial, rationalization, and projection. The evidence continues to mount, making it impossible for the alcoholic to ignore the developing problem. The family will no longer accept the blame. Their confrontations become stronger. And as the alcoholic begins to process all the information, the reaction of fear is to be expected.

Fear results from the certainty of knowing that something is not normal. It is also produced by the uncertainty of the cause of the problem and of what to do. The alcoholic becomes afraid that he or she may be going crazy or may end up on skid row. The alcoholic is afraid for the future and afraid for life. He or she may sense the havoc within the family. The awareness of the family problems produces a fear of being left alone. The alcoholic may also fear that the entire family may be destroyed.

The fifth psychological reaction is *anger*. Anger—intense anger—is an emotion common to all alcoholics. Some experts say it is the intense anger that causes the heavy drinking, but in reality, it is the alcoholism that causes the anger. The alcoholic becomes more aware that the problem is real and that it does involve the drinking. The evidence continues to pour in as the person is confronted with the consequences of the drinking. Accepting society's view of alcoholism, the alcoholic feels weak due to the inability to control the problem. The phrase "I should be able to control this!" continues to torment the alcoholic. Family members, friends, and business associates repeat the same message: "You should be able to handle this. You must take control." The more unmanageable the problem becomes, the greater the intensity of the rage.

Not knowing how the alcoholism developed, the alcoholic comes to the conclusion that "I have caused this myself." You can imagine how an executive who has had many successes becomes so frustrated and angry with the discovery of a problem that cannot be brought under control by personal effort. The anger is intense, and it spews out onto all those near the alcoholic; they in turn confront the person with the intensity of their own emotions. This anger is enhanced by the toxicity in the brain. The fear of the confrontations and outbursts of rage leave the alcoholic with an overwhelming feeling of helplessness. As the anger is stuffed inside and the helpless feelings grow, depression overtakes the alcoholic.

Depression has been termed "a temper tantrum turned inward." In the case of the alcoholic, this seems appropriate. The unresolved rage seeps into every aspect of the psychological economy, leaving behind a depressed mind.

These deep periods of depression produce more reasons to drink. And as large amounts of the depressant drug alcohol are consumed, the depression darkens. This is not a depression common to most people. Its pain, increased by toxicity and emotional augmentation, far exceeds that of normal depression. It is living life in the pits.

For the alcoholic in this stage of the progression, life seems to be slipping away. The system of denial that has been constructed and reinforced over the years, combined with the devastating depression, leaves the alcoholic paralyzed and stagnant. As the depression lingers, the drinking becomes a constant companion. When the alcoholic does briefly stop drinking, the depression is so great that he or she must drink for relief. Those around the alcoholic, seeing the magnitude of the problem while drinking and even more problems when the drinking stops, also become paralyzed. Vibrant, active families, once involved with life at its best, are now engulfed in sadness.

The paralysis in both the family and the alcoholic assists in the *deterioration of self-image* in the alcoholic. The self-image deteriorates because, after many futile attempts to reform, the alcoholic begins to believe "I don't have what it takes." He or she feels "no good," weak, and characterless. After losing family, friends, and job, the alcoholic finds it impossible to rediscover the real person of worth beneath the drinking. All the willpower available is mustered, and with each failure, the self-image deteriorates even more. The alcoholic comes to maintain only unhealthy relationships. The only friends are those who are inferior or at least appear inferior. It is an indication that the alcoholic is nearing bottom.

The natural reaction to the deterioration of self-image is a total *personality distortion*. The individual is nothing like the person who drank moderately years before. Accompanying the destruction of the self-image is the deterioration of former values. Things that were once priorities become unimportant. Those things that were esteemed perish in the struggle to survive. The life of the alcoholic turns into a Jekyll-and-Hyde existence. The mind, so affected by the chemical and the psychological reactions, becomes an unpredictable mass of contradictions. Repeatedly the alcoholic moves from "Mr. or Mrs. Wonderful" back into destructive behaviors that hurt others in his or her life. It is common for alcoholics to have periods when all the thoughtful and romantic acts that could be imagined are carried out, or at the office the alcoholic may for a brief time do the work of two or three people. But the flurry of activity ends in another bout of predictably uncontrolled drinking and destructive behavior. The more productive and wonderful the behavior during the good times, the greater are the false hopes, dashed once again.

The final two psychological reactions are *arrested maturity* and *infantile behavior*. Because of the reactions that have preceded them, the ability to deal with emotions has stopped. Emotions are dealt with by running from people or to more alcohol and other chemicals. Life for the alcoholic is a vain attempt to cope and a constant search for relief. Compensation for failure and attempts to change spiral into a mass of unmanageable consequences. Concepts of maturity like honesty, patience, and humility disappear from the alcoholic's life. Personal growth gives way to the destruction of maturity all through the late stages of the disease.

The disease leaves the alcoholic with a very low stress tolerance. The slightest problem or discomfort can set off a chain of demanding and defiant behavior that would be expected from a child but is unacceptable from an adult. Easily upset, the alcoholic is avoided by all those who know that just on the other side of the calmness of the moment lurks a scene full of negative emotions and pain. Those close to the alcoholic stand in complete disgust as they witness the exaggerated reactions to minor problems. The effects of the alcohol are clearer than ever. They are amplified by the alcoholic's regression into infantile and immature behavior.

The physical symptoms in the progression begin the destruction. The psychological reactions thrust the alcoholic even deeper into a chasm of inability to change. The progression leaves in its wake a person totally unaware that change can occur. If change were to occur, it could not happen without help from others. But because of the alcoholic's distorted interpretations of all that has happened, he or she knows nothing but aloneness. The interpretations are the elements that keep the alcoholic from the world of recovery.

SPIRITUAL INTERPRETATION

The following spiritual interpretations could be called the "killer list" in the progression of the problem. It is in this area that the spiritual life of the alcoholic is severely damaged, and a total separation from other people and God results. Because the alcoholic feels that the physical symptoms and the psychological reactions are self-inflicted, the set of spiritual interpretations are deadly. Society convinces the alcoholic that all the problems are caused by inadequacy, moral degradation, or weakness and the alcoholic's inability to cope with life. Because society's lack of understanding promotes the stigma of alcoholism, the alcoholic ends up in total isolation.

Guilt is the first emotion in the list of interpretations. In alcoholics undergoing treatment, guilt seems to prevail over all the other emotions. Although the anger flares from time to time, guilt infects every interaction. Probably one of the greatest values of treatment is the discovery for each alcoholic that he or she is not alone in guilt. The guilt is moored in the belief that all the problems have been self-inflicted. Society's indictment is that the alcoholic has chosen his or her malady. The guilt is a major contributor to inaction on the part of the alcoholic.

Coupled with the guilt is *shame* for being an alcoholic. The alcoholic feels guilt for not changing and shame for having the label of alcoholism; this is, of course, heightened by the stigma. The shame and the guilt produce deadly thoughts that acceptance by self, others, and God is impossible. This causes the person to hide and avoid people like a leper; the condition is viewed as unpardonable.

Remorse is a natural companion to the guilt and shame. The remorse comes as the alcoholic reflects incessantly back on all that has happened as a result of drinking. The alcoholic finds himself or herself in deep sorrow, continuing to wallow in a past that cannot be changed. He or she is deeply contrite over the hurt inflicted on others. The guilt, shame, and remorse build a cage of self-pity that destroys the ability of the alcoholic to see any hope for change.

These three interpretations of the progression separate the alcoholic from help as he or she ends up feeling total *alienation*. The alienation prevents the alcoholic from getting close to anyone, especially anyone with insight into the problem. Because the alcoholic hates what is on the inside, there is an attempt to protect that from everyone else. Of course, this also leads to the self-hatred that causes greater alienation from God. The alcoholic, believing he or she has caused it all, thinks if there is a God, He would not care about someone so guilty. This cuts off all spiritual growth. The alcoholic avoids people, discussions, and places that have anything to do with spirituality, God, or church. The alcoholic, alienated from God and others, is left to suffer alone.

But the alcoholic cannot recover alone. While help is needed for support and direction, the alcoholic is alienated from anyone who could help. Each new encounter becomes a repeated process of sizing up and rejecting. "They don't really care." "He hasn't been through what I've been through." "How could you help someone like me?" All become the battle cries of continued alienation. One by one the alcoholic figures out some excuse to push everyone out of his or her life.

As the alcoholic isolates himself or herself from the world and God, *insecurity* grows. The alcoholic, out of relationships with other people and in no relationship with God, feels misplaced in life—as if everyone else fits but the alcoholic. For some the insecurity is so great that it leads to paranoia. He or she not only feels misplaced but imagines that God or other people are out to destroy what person there is left.

The alcoholic, with no relationship and no sense of purpose or direction, is overcome by *worthlessness*, feeling contemptible and deserving of failure. For some there is financial bankruptcy, but for every alcoholic, at the end of a long progression in a futile battle to overcome the alcoholism, there is spiritual bankruptcy. The alcoholic, at the end of a wasted and ruined desert of years, feels deserted in the midst of a life with no meaning.

The incredible emptiness and the belief that all the problems have been self-inflicted sets up a whole chain of *reactions to punish self*. The alcoholic feels deserving of failure and consequently will set himself or herself up to fail. If there is someone who exerts an unhealthy influence on the alcoholic's life, there is a tremendous tendency to become involved in a relationship with that person. It is sad, but very common, for those in the most destructive stages of alcoholism to be attracted to each other. The cliché "Misery loves company" is true. If there are two people downtrodden by guilt and set up to fail, they will probably find each other. The association will frequently reinforce old behaviors and prevent the development of new insights.

This problem of self-inflicted failure also manifests itself in business deals that are destined to fail or in accepting positions too difficult to handle. These new jobs that are beyond the scope of the person always end up with either a resignation or dismissal. When you hear of all the problems and failures, it is hard to believe that so many dreadful things could happen to one person. The only way it could is for the person to be unconsciously working at self-punishment. That person is rigged to fail. The guilt over a devastated life drives the alcoholic toward destruction.

The last of the interpretations of life for the alcoholic is total *despair*. The alcoholic now views life as a purposeless struggle, a road going nowhere. In this despair, many alcoholics succeed at suicide. It is often said that alcoholism is a slow form of suicide, but that is inaccurate. The use of alcohol eventually becomes a means to survive; it is a poor choice, but it is an attempt to hold on to whatever is left. At the end of the progression, the alcoholic finally considers the suicide option.

The progression, 100 percent of the time, ends in death from disease, an accident, suicide, or total insanity. It is said that nothing can totally destroy a life as effectively as alcoholism. It has the ability to destroy every area of the individual's life. Every area of hope or potential turns into sadness, but the sadness does not center on the alcoholic alone. The family and friends also become victims of the devastation. They are dragged through the symptoms, reactions, and interpretations with the alcoholic. It's not just the alcoholic who needs recovery after a life of despair; every family member needs help, too.

Recovery is not simple. It certainly does not occur just from stopping the drinking. And even treatment at times will not be effective in initiating recovery. The reason is the collection of deadly spiritual interpretations—the "killer list." These spiritual interpretations will remain unless the alcoholic takes great effort to resolve them. It is puzzling to many that some alcoholics remain miserable after years of not drinking. It is very likely due to the lack of healing in the spiritual dimension. Quality of life improves at the point of spiritual resolution.

The resolution of the spiritual interpretations begins with accepting the disease concept of alcoholism. The alcoholic accepts

that the alcoholism is a result of a body that processed the alcohol abnormally and not of a self-inflicted motivation toward
destruction. If this concept is not accepted, the alcoholic's life
will veer off into one of two directions. One is back to drinking
to escape the guilt for what has happened. The other direction
is away from drinking but toward compensating for all that has
happened. Compensation involves the development of workaholism, religious fanaticism, or any of a number of behaviors
that destroy the individual's ability to grow. It is common to see
the alcoholic vacillate between the two directions. There are
times of abstinence and extreme efforts to make up for the past,
followed by an eventual return to drinking. This roller coaster
of pseudorecovery and relapse is just as deadly as continued
drinking, and it is certainly more destructive to the family. The
alcoholic and the family will remain stagnant and devoid of any
growth. Spiritual recovery pulls the alcoholic out of the repeti-
tion of guilt and compensation. It allows the growth of maturity
and stability in the alcoholic.

In addition to accepting alcoholism as a chronic, progressive
physiological disease, the alcoholic must also allow God to forgive all the things that have happened during the progression of
the disease. This is really the beginning of spiritual recovery for
the alcoholic. Without forgiveness, the alienation from God and
other people will continue, and the feelings of worthlessness
and despair will continue, eventually controlling the person's
whole life again.

Spiritual recovery restores the alcoholic's sense of value and
worth and is responsible for long-term recovery instead of short-
term results. Spiritual recovery is greatly needed for the alcoholic, and yet few people recover spiritually. If this area of
recovery is not achieved, the alcoholic will never fully regain a
"normal" life-style. He or she will retain a distorted self-concept and a lack of purpose and meaning in life. Whether drinking or abstaining, the alcoholic is not in recovery unless the
spiritual interpretations are resolved.

It is important to identify where in the progression the spiritual problems began. They began when the tolerance went up
and the emotional augmentation set in. Looking at the progression, many have concluded that the results, both psychological
and spiritual, are the cause. This is because the initial stages are
invisible to most. In viewing the results of alcoholism as the

cause, attempts at recovery occur out of sequence. The proper sequence is physical, mental, and *then* spiritual. Reversing the order only adds frustration to the alcoholic's life.

Of course, there are those who have made a remarkable recovery through some initial experience or awakening. This rare occurrence is called *spontaneous recovery*. But there is no guarantee that this will happen for every alcoholic any more than there is a guarantee of an instant healing in every cancer patient. It is unwise to attempt results based on exceptions rather than on a logical plan that has worked for thousands of alcoholics. A quick fix most likely will not correct what took years to develop.

Finally, in putting the physical, mental, and spiritual aspects of alcoholism in perspective, note three main points. First, the progression will proceed through all three areas to the point of death or insanity unless recovery is initiated. Second, because of a brain physiologically damaged from toxicity, the alcoholic's mind does not function normally. If it did, the alcoholic would be able to identify the problem, stop drinking, and start recovery. It is irrational for anyone to wait for an alcoholic magically to decide one day to stop drinking and start recovery. The alcoholic will eventually reach that point, but it will be after the consequences of the drinking are so great that no other choice remains. Third, the person closest to the alcoholic is the person most likely to assist the alcoholic in initiating recovery. The action to be taken should not be in the area of resolving psychological conflicts or spiritual interpretations first. Efforts should be focused on physiological healing initially. This involves giving the body time to heal. Once detoxification occurs, it is vital that the alcoholic be supported through the resolution of both the psychological and spiritual progressions.

Remember that the alcoholic does not choose to be alcoholic. It is the body that reacts differently to the chemical. This difference in the physiological makeup of the alcoholic is to blame. Once this concept can be accepted, a world of freedom awaits those who are trapped by alcoholism and the stigma that is supported by a society that does not understand.

CHAPTER NINE

SIX PERSONALITIES OF AN ALCOHOLIC

I opened this book with Stephanie's story, which presented in dramatic form the progress of addiction up to the point of deciding to seek treatment. Subsequent chapters explored the nature of alcoholism and the alcoholic progression, with the material, I hope, made more immediate by having seen it demonstrated in Stephanie's life. Sam Jorgenson's story takes the progression further, into and through recovery, and will both give another perspective on the progression and serve as an introduction to the many facets of recovery.

Sam Jorgenson had never touched a drop of alcohol. He had purposely delayed the time when he would consume his first drink. He was only sixteen years old, and he decided it was something that should best be done when he was older. But like most adolescents, he was under pressure to drink from friends and all of society.

Sam had remained an abstainer while his friends began drinking as young as ages ten and eleven. He had done so because, to him, alcohol was not just a chemical in a bottle, but a force that had already affected his life dramatically. That effect was the impact of alcohol on his parents. Sam's mom and dad were living together, but they had been mentally and emotionally divorced for a long time. Sam's dad was an alcoholic. Sam had watched his dad emerge from a warm, caring man who controlled his drinking to an unpredictable recluse who barricaded himself from his family and the world with thousands of bottles of alcohol. Over the years, the more control of the family his father lost because of drinking, the more control his mother had gained. Throughout his entire childhood, he had been in constant turmoil over his troublesome home life. Sam had watched his mother grab more and more responsibilities as his dad slipped further and further into a world no one in the family understood. Eventually his mother became a living paradox—in total control of everything except for the father's drinking and the father.

It was lack of understanding that motivated Sam to remain an abstainer. He could not figure out how such a seemingly harmless substance had totally destroyed his dad's identity and self-respect. He withstood the pressure from friends to drink because of the tension and stress he experienced at home. It had made him afraid of alcohol, and yet he was also intensely fascinated by it. Inside he knew that once he drank, he would be able to control it. He felt that, unlike his father, he would not succumb to the powerful force behind the drink. But he was not sure. The insecurity he felt over his family and the effects of alcohol on it provided an extra incentive to choose not to drink.

Sam, like many young people his age, was very shy. In a large crowd or in a small group of friends, his words were forced, and as he spoke, he questioned everything he said. He would mull over every interaction and conclude that he had probably said the wrong thing or that someone else could have said it better. His shyness was normal for his age, but it went beyond what his peers experienced. He felt inferior because his dad had been so negative to him all his life. His dad, in an effort to build himself up, had constantly put Sam down. Nothing Sam did was good enough. The impact of this was significant for Sam's relationships with others.

Sam felt awkward around his friends, adults, and especially girls. He was very naïve and inexperienced when it came to developing a relationship with the opposite sex. The amazing thing was Sam's popularity with the girls. He was the fastest running back on the school's football team in his junior year. In the eyes of many, he was a true hometown hero. Although he was unsophisticated about the ways of the world, he certainly had the eyes of a small portion of the world on him. No one would have guessed that beneath the handsome exterior of a fine athlete and student was a growing apprehension about life that thrust Sam into the emotional extremes of adolescence. The facade of complete security and competence hid a deep emptiness within him.

In Sam's small town, most of the kids went to the Baptist church, where a youth director coordinated activities for the young people. Sam liked going to church because it was a safe place. There the kids were a little more open about expressing feelings of inadequacies and sharing the pains of growing up. It was also a place where he and some of his friends could go without the pressure to drink. Everyone in that church and most of the townspeople marveled at Sam. "How could such a fine young man come from such a tragic home where there was no father to set an example?" Sam knew what people thought, for some had even expressed it to him. It actually motivated him to do better. He would not let anything derail his path toward success. He knew of his own potential, and he wanted to make the best of it.

Back then, Sam was one big mass of potential—the All-American Boy growing up with all of the normal pressures and anxieties of teenagers. Sam Jorgenson, a nervous, uptight adolescent, seemed to be on top of the world. He couldn't dance, but on the football field, he could move with the grace and style of a star player. It was hard for him to make conversation, but a lot of the girls just wanted a word or two with him. He was good in sports, earned good grades, and was known as an all-around good boy. It appeared that if anyone would succeed out of that small high school in that small town, it would be Sam Jorgenson.

Years later Sam looked back on those uneasy but exciting days of his youth. For a long time he brooded over what might have happened had he stayed on course toward success. He had to break loose from the paralyzing trap of the "if onlys." "If only I had remained an abstainer." "If only my family had been different." "If only," the two words that are the steps downward toward regret. Sam Jorgenson, like his dad, eventually experienced the devastating progression of alcoholism. He felt great remorse as he longed to relive those days when he never drank, when life was full of potential. Eventually he grew to accept that an alcoholic can never return to that first personality stage called the *abstainer*. Sam's eventual recovery allowed him to forge ahead and leave the wasteful regret behind. But for a long time it was for Sam, as it is for many alcoholics, a roadblock to his recovery.

Sam had a great senior year in football, and academically as well, and was awarded an athletic scholarship at a major university. In the fall, he went off to continue his triumphs.

College proved to be an exciting time for eighteen-year-old

Sam Jorgenson. Although he was only ninety miles away from his hometown, he felt like he was in a different universe. Thousands of people were running around looking just as confused and excited as he was. No one from his high school had come to this college. He did not know a soul, and for the first time in years, no one knew him, either, except the coaches who had recruited him. He was a nobody who would have to fight hard for the recognition he had obtained back home—the recognition that had helped him combat the constant feelings of inferiority and ineptitude.

During Sam's first year of college, something happened that would eventually prove to be the most significant event of his life. Sam took his first drink. The pressure to drink was quite strong at college and intensified when Sam pledged a fraternity. It seemed that everyone considered drinking a vital part of fraternity life. Sam's pledge brothers told him that if he expected to make it, he had better learn to drink. They told him it was just unnatural for a guy not to drink at all. The more they talked, the more Sam realized that the day of his first drink was getting closer. He wanted to belong, and it became apparent to him that the only way he could feel part of the group and be accepted was to drink with the crowd. No one in his life was encouraging him not to drink.

The big event occurred at his fraternity's fall formal dance. The fall formal was an overnight event in another town where everyone supposedly had a great time at a very dressy dinner and dance. Of course, many of the attendees were so intoxicated that they never remembered whether or not they had a great time. Fall formals overflowed with alcohol, and Sam's fraternity drank more than others. For much of the weekend the young men were totally out of control. Drunkenness was the ulterior motive behind going away; the formal was just a good excuse.

So it was in the setting of a drunken fall formal that Sam Jorgenson left the abstainer behind forever and became a drinker. When it happened, he was in the presence of one of his fraternity's "little sisters." They had met while he was pledging and had become good friends. They felt safe with each other, and when Sam asked, she accepted the invitation to the formal. By her side, in the middle of the Grand Ballroom, Sam took his first drink. He walked over to the bartender (he could legally drink at eighteen) and asked for a rum-and-Coke. The bartender met his request and handed over a tall glass of cold Coke with rum. Sam walked back over to Kathy, put the drink to his lips, and drank it all in one big gulp. The drink made him feel warm inside. After a minute or two, he grabbed Kathy around the waist and whisked her off to dance. And dance they did! Sam had never danced so well in his entire life. In fact, he had hardly danced in his entire life. But tonight was different; he danced and he loved dancing. Kathy thought he was outstanding also. So for the next hour, Sam and Kathy stayed on the floor dancing, talking, and growing closer.

Finally they sat down at a table with four other couples, and when Kathy asked Sam to get her a drink, he did. And he got one for himself also. He felt good and relaxed with the others at the table; telling funny stories, talking football, and just being himself came easily. He discovered something that he had suspected for a long time. Alcohol really did work. It had turned a naïve, awkward college freshman into a fanciful dancer, a fearless conversationalist, and a social genius. He did not become wildly drunk or intoxicated; he just felt relaxed and warmly accepted. He was a part of the group—he belonged. He wondered why it had taken him so long to reach this point of drinking. He could see no harm in what he had done. And he looked forward to the next opportunity to drink again.

That night, Sam Jorgenson began drinking for the same reason everyone else drinks: to feel an effect. In the beginning, what a person wants alcohol to do has a lot to do with what it actually does. The effect of alcohol is self-generated to a large degree. It temporarily picks up the depressed and calms down the agitated. Often the results of drink are more influenced by the mind of the drinker than the alcohol in the drink. For most people, the combination of the attitude, the setting, and the alcohol serves to fulfill the expectation. That's why there has been such a fascination with alcohol for thousands of years. If there were not something magical about this chemical, there would never have been so much attention given to different ways to produce it. At eighteen, Sam Jorgenson discovered the magic.

For Sam, his first drinking experience was a pleasurable one. There would be many more to follow. He never forgot those fun times associated with his early drinking. Whether he drank with buddies or with girlfriends, the memory was pleasant. He always remembered that in the beginning, his drinking changed his personality a bit; but not in a bad or negative way. He remembered the positive changes. When he drank, he was more relaxed and at ease. He could talk, dance, and be sociable more easily. In those beginning days of drinking, he was very cautious. He rarely drank enough to get drunk. And he never drove after he had been drinking. He never forgot how responsible he was and how much fun he had.

Sam did well throughout college, making the dean's list most semesters and again establishing himself as a football hero. He and Kathy were married the summer before his senior year. Their last year of college together was a great way to start a marriage. They had tremendous support from their friends and family. Sam's dad had died his junior year, and the insurance and inheritance were large enough so that money was no problem. For Sam and Kathy Jorgenson, it was the best of times. They had plenty of friends and plenty of fun. Sam had made a perfect transition from the "model" young man to part of a "model" couple.

Sam handled every area of his life, and especially success, very well. To Kathy, he was just "good old Sam," even though he was often in the spotlight. His drinking remained what appeared to be an insignificant part of his life. He drank a beer or two with the guys during the week, and every other weekend or so, there would be a fraternity party, or some of the athletes would have a little get-together around a keg of beer. Sam was inconspicuous as a drinker. While others regularly became drunk, he was always able to hold his alcohol. His tolerance had gradually increased beyond that of his friends. For some reason, he was able to drink a lot of alcohol and not feel the effects of it, like the other guys. While they might drink three or four glasses of beer and lose control, Sam could drink two six-packs over an evening and have no problems. If there was anything unique about his drinking, it was not the effect it had on him, but rather that he could drink so much with so little effect. Unlike the very early days of drinking, he rarely felt the changes that had been so intriguing during his first drinks.

Success continued to be the track for Sam. In his senior year of college, he signed on with a pro team and won professional football's "Rookie of the Year" award. It did not take long for him to receive nationally the recognition that he had once obtained in his hometown. He and Kathy were again in the spotlight, and they enjoyed it. And while the spotlight was on, they started their family. Each year for four years, Sam and Kathy had a new baby. Sam's career continued to be successful. As a family of six, they had access to an unlimited number of opportunities because of Sam's large salary. To most people, Sam and Kathy had it made. Fame, fortune, and a wonderful family were all components of a dream come true.

After ten years of marriage, the dream was not without its times of trouble and disappointments. In the midst of having it made, a problem began to worry Kathy. Sam was no longer a pillar of emotional stability. His warm and loving nature was at times anything but warm and loving. He was frequently irritated and angered by very trivial occurrences. As the years went by, the problem became worse. His irritation would mount into a fit of rage. His rage would grow until finally he would put a fist through a wall, throw something, or run out of the house to escape. Kathy's worry was for herself and for her children. It was obvious that they were being affected. They did not run to their father when he came home; they waited to find out his mood. Both Kathy and the kids were afraid of what might happen during the next fit of anger. Sam's drinking had increased in both frequency and quantity. Drinking was a regular part of his life. Every day after practice, he would have four or five drinks in the evening, and every weekend there would be a party, a dinner out, or the two of them alone at home with a lot of drinking on Sam's part. His tolerance had increased to the point where Kathy thought the alcohol never fazed him. She could never accuse him of being drunk. While he was drinking, he was under control. It was the day after that caused the problem. That was when it was almost unbearable to be with Sam. The progression of events became very predictable.

During the off season, Sam drank more than when he was playing, and he drank most on the weekends. If Friday night was a time of heavy consumption, then Saturday was a predictable fiasco. To Kathy it was as if he were in withdrawal from the alcohol. His personality would make a total reversal. He would be extremely agitated and irritable. At times he would even be quite nauseated, but for the most part, he was just very anxious and uncomfortable. He acted as if he did not care for Kathy or the children. He would focus totally on himself and his own discomfort. It became the job of Kathy and the four children to make him comfortable. If anyone stepped out of line, it would mean another burst of anger or a trip to the refrigerator for a beer. The first beer would lead to almost a case of beer in one day.

Kathy would start each Saturday with a lecture to the kids about "Daddy's rough week" and how important it was to be quiet and not disturb him. And they would all try very hard to be good and not get Dad riled up. But between the four of them, it was an impossible assignment. No matter how hard they tried, they always failed it. Someone would play the television too loud or scream or do something that would wake Sam up in a state of distress. Many mornings, he would stomp from the bedroom directly to the kitchen. On the way he would rattle off a guilt-inflicting oration about his need for rest, his need for respect, and his need for quiet. In the kitchen he would satisfy his greatest need, his need for alcohol.

Something very strange was happening at the Jorgensons' house. (Yet it happens in almost every home of every alcoholic.) Sam was drinking more and more and acting very strange. It was phenomenal how he had made the transition into unpredictable and intolerable behavior. Kathy was denying that the problem was getting worse. She wrote it off to an athlete's increasing insecurity over aging. But the kids were not denying the problem. They were beginning to accept some responsibility for it. They knew there must be a reason for such a bizarre change in their father. They were starting to think that if they were just a little better or closer to perfect, Dad would not need to drink so much or become so angry. Everyone in the family was more aware of the problem each day. As the reality of it grew, no one was allowed to discuss it. This strange phenomenon was to be avoided as a topic of conversation at all costs. Dad's anger or Dad's drinking were to be ignored. Even at its worst, when it was impossible to be ignored, it had to be eliminated from all discussions.

Sam was definitely different. He was growing older and more distant and notably more unpredictable. It seemed that the only thing that made him appear normal was to drink alcohol. If he was drinking, he appeared more comfortable and easier to deal with. At times he was his old self. It was those mornings after that were becoming more and more frequent and impossible to endure. He made those mornings extremely hard on the family.

No one knew what to do, so they did nothing—except live in constant fear.

Sam played football for ten years before retiring. He had been fortunate to have a good manager who handled his money. When his ten years in pro ball were up, Sam was financially secure for life. He did not need to work at all; he could live off his investments. When he left the field for the last time, he did so proudly. He left a winner. With his money, he set up a small public relations firm for which his fame was the chief asset. It did well and enabled his wealth to grow even more. His drinking problem grew also. His thinking was very confused. He could not concentrate very long on any one subject. Or even worse, he would go off on a tangent and talk for hours about some meaningless event or topic. He would mull it over in his mind and repeat his comments out loud again and again. This behavior was not only confusing, but annoying to others. It produced a whole new fear in Kathy, that Sam might lose control completely, that he was going crazy and would never be the same.

Sam's memory was also being affected. He could tell you exactly where he was twenty years ago when John F. Kennedy was assassinated, but he could not remember a discussion about vacation plans from two days earlier. The short-term memory seemed to be destroyed. It was as if events just were not registering. Of course this affected his business. He could not make good decisions, nor could he remember the decisions he had made. Employees at his firm did not stay very long.

His emotions were grossly distorted. He was either intensely agitated, almost manic, or deeply depressed. His mood swings were incredible from one hour to the next. Whatever the mood, it was obvious that he was not in control of his emotions; they were in control of him. He was constantly battling the extremes of his feelings. It was as if two people lived inside one man.

In addition to his thinking, memory, and emotional problems, Sam was also losing judgment. He seemed to hire the wrong people, get involved with the wrong projects. Failure piled on top of failure. His values appeared either to be disintegrating or at least shifting. He began to cheat on his taxes and even lie to his friends and family. No one could depend on him. His decisions—usually poor ones—frequently contradicted one another. His own inconsistency embarrassed him. That dean's-list mind had lost its ability to function; it had moved from the asset column to the liability column.

Sam's willpower was also gone. He could not refuse a drink. He had lost his ability to be in control or to take control. Something had happened to make a very powerful man powerless over alcohol. It had also rendered him powerless in all other areas of life. His brain was sick from all the alcohol, and yet no one was doing anything to help. Kathy had seen counselors, but they had concluded that Sam was either schizophrenic or manic-depressive. They convinced her that counseling could clear up those mental problems and eliminate the need to drink. Confused, Kathy did not know what the problem was. But whatever it was, it had produced a totally different Sam Jorgenson.

Life was miserable for Sam. The more he tried to gain control, the more control he lost. Everything he did increased his alienation from others. No one could stand to be with him very long. Sam's world became filled with anger and resentment because he could not regain control of his family, his business, or his life. He had no idea how to stop his downward spiral. And the further down his spirit plummeted, the greater his anger at himself and the world around him grew. As his drinking caused more problems, the problems caused more drinking. His only goal was somehow to hope and survive. Everyday survival became increasingly doubtful.

The effects of Sam's drinking were obvious to everyone around him. However, his denial was so strong that he could not see it. As his control over his life had weakened, so had his ability to control his drinking. The more he drank, the more he lost control, and the more those around him pleaded for him to stop drinking. They could no longer sit back and watch him suffer and afflict everyone around with pain and frustration. He could no longer drink as much as in days past. His tolerance for the chemical had dropped, and at times one drink was intoxicating. What used to produce no effect would send him into wild drunkenness or a solemn stupor.

One day Kathy had finally had enough. She was convinced that he had to stop drinking. She believed it was the only answer. She told Sam that she loved him, cared about him, and wanted the best for him, but she would not stay with him if he continued to drink. He had to decide between the alcohol and her. Both could not exist together. Sam loved Kathy greatly, and, out of fear of losing her, he agreed to stop drinking. He promised that if she would stay and stick by him, he would never touch another drop. Kathy hoped that this was the answer and that they would be able to patch up the personal wounds and rebuild their family. She did not think it was too late. But as Kathy was to discover, stopping the drinking was not the total answer. It would take more than just life without a bottle to rebuild a relationship and a family.

Alcoholics who stop drinking but don't start recovery are said to be *dry* rather than *sober*. Life for a dry alcoholic is usually as horrible as the late stages of alcoholism. For Sam, the dry stage was more miserable than the others. He, too, had hoped the pieces would somehow fall in place with the cessation of the drinking, but it just did not happen. If anything, the pieces became more scattered. His life was a greater mess than before. When he stopped drinking, he set in motion the progression of a whole new set of problems.

Sam had a lot tied up in his attempt to stop drinking. It was his last-ditch effort to regain control of his life. His wife, his job, and his family hung in the balance. The pressure to regain control was something he felt every waking minute. He had never attempted anything so difficult or painful in his entire life. He wanted to call upon the past resources that had helped to make him successful. Anything he could do on his own, he was willing to do, in desperation to stay off alcohol. An hour did not go by without him thinking of what he could do to prevent taking another drink.

Sam was obsessed. He was obsessed with alcohol, drinking, and his need to succeed at stopping. His entire ego was at stake as he feared the failure that was almost guaranteed. Saddled with the guilt from what had happened due to the drinking and from not stopping years earlier, he felt spent and weak but determined to fight to quit drinking.

As a result, Sam began to overcompensate for all that he felt. He tightened the reins on family spending. He demanded the checkbook back from his wife and would not allow any checks to be written without his permission. He wanted to control the money, the budget, and all the finances. He stated that he was finally going to reassert himself as head of the family. He demanded to be in control. But his overbearing control was frustrating for the family. He bore down on each member, driving each one further away from him than the drinking had.

His obsession also prompted him to exert control over those who worked for him. He implemented a system of quotas that was unreasonable and unacceptable to his account representatives in the public relations firm. They confronted him and threatened to leave if he did not let up on his demands. But their threats only made him more demanding. The harder he worked to control the agency, the greater others resisted him. Employees left because the pressure was unbearable.

Through all this, thoughts of drinking and the need to not drink repeatedly invaded Sam's mind. He was driven to thoughts of alcohol and the relief he wanted, which it could provide. Sam did not know it, but he was addicted to alcohol. And although he had stopped the drinking, the power of addiction was greater than ever. He found himself in an overwhelming state of obsession. No matter how hard he tried, the thoughts of alcohol and drinking drove other thoughts out of his mind. Every day without alcohol increased the intensity of the obsession with it.

He was also obsessed with guilt for the past and anxiety and fear for the future. Recurring nightmares from reliving the past and dread over what might happen if all control was lost prevented him from focusing on the present. His life was only a state of illusion. He thought he was in control, but was instead a victim of addiction. Every reaction was due to alcohol's grip on his mind and body. He tried to figure out what he should do in his determination to handle the problem on his own. But all his attempts and overcompensation left him angry and engulfed in his own misery.

The effort not to drink paralyzed him. His life had produced some deep, infected wounds that required treatment, not a series of Band-Aids. Kathy was more depressed than ever. His stopping drinking had been her hope for a normal life, but the longer Sam resisted alcohol, the worse their relationship grew. Sam had become more irrational than when he drank. Now he was experiencing all sorts of compulsive behaviors. He ate almost all of the time and had gained thirty pounds. For the first time in his life, he smoked. And in contrast to his efforts to control the money, he would go on spending sprees and compulsively buy worthless, needless items. He was more out of control than ever, but in his thick web of delusions, he thought he was doing better. He continued to think that each day without alcohol was a victory.

He flaunted his ability to not drink in front of everyone he knew. He was obnoxious, arranging meetings in bars and shouting, "Just water for me!" In restaurants he would beg Kathy to order wine and display to the waiter his grand ritual of turning his own glass over. If anyone came to the house, it was an invitation for him to display his control. He would serve drinks from his own bar and make sure everyone knew that he did not need to drink. Again, he was paralyzed and obsessed with his alcoholic thinking.

One day Sam came home from work to find a note from Kathy. It simply stated that she would be home later and asked him to fix himself dinner. For some irrational reason, this enraged Sam. He could not believe she would be so inconsiderate as to be gone when he came home. He could not believe she wanted him to fix his own dinner. He told himself that she was just trying to infuriate him and make him miserable. He felt as if she wanted him to drink again and was setting him up to fail. In his rage, he flew out the door to seek revenge for what he perceived as an open act of aggression. He drove straight to his favorite bar, slammed down a ten-dollar bill, and demanded a pitcher of beer. He grabbed the pitcher, hoisted it, and within one minute had drunk the entire contents. Yes, he was drinking again, but he felt he deserved to. As the effects of the alcohol set in, Sam's intense anger turned to sorrowful remorse. He knew he had compounded failure with another failure. He cried as he slumped before the bartender, who had watched his problem progress to this deep level of depression.

The man behind the bar summoned a cab for Sam. Both Kathy's and Sam's cabs arrived at the house at the same time. Kathy helped him through the door, and in that dark, gray, hopeless moment, they both knew they could not help themselves. Kathy could not help Sam, and Sam was beyond helping himself. Kathy told Sam that something had to be done and she was calling a treatment center for help. To her, enough time and effort had been spent futilely; a wasted life could be tolerated no longer.

Kathy phoned the local Council on Alcoholism to ask for help. Given several alternatives, the counselor guided her toward the choice of an inpatient hospital setting.

That evening Sam was admitted to a unit for the treatment of alcoholism and drug abuse. It was finally, after a life of dim hope, a beginning. It was Sam and Kathy's hope for a move out of the world of drinking and into the world of sobriety. It was Sam's first move toward acquiring the sixth personality stage of the alcoholic, the sober one.

The treatment for alcoholism was a life-changing experience for Sam, Kathy, and their four children. Sam was not the only one who was treated. Everyone was a part of the recovery process. It was intense, at times extremely emotionally painful, but every thread and fiber of the program offered hope for understanding and hope for a better life. Hope had eluded Sam and Kathy for years, but during treatment, it felt real. They had finally met people who knew the source of the problem and exactly what to do about it. They no longer felt alone.

For Sam, treatment was very confusing in the beginning. He found himself with people who had the same problem but varying degrees of motivation to change. Some talked as if they were just hanging in until their discharge date, when they would return to the bottle. Others spent time trying to figure out how they could drink while still in treatment. Fortunately for Sam, he was placed in a room with a man who had been in treatment for three weeks, gone through the doubting and game playing, and developed a desire to do whatever it took to not drink again. He was a strong role model for Sam. He would help Sam develop a plan to ensure he had the best chance possible of staying sober.

Sam's second day of treatment began with a morning meditation time with all the other patients. During meditation, the leader talked about turning things over to a higher power. "Let go and let God" was the message of the day, but the leader also stressed that each individual must do his or her own part. Everyone must work to grow more open and honest and in the process accept the limitations of humanity. The more the acceptance, the greater our ability to allow a higher power to control what we cannot. The leader explained that for most alcoholics, there is great alienation from God. The guilt deteriorates and prevents development of the spiritual aspect of life. As the progression intensifies, the alcoholic becomes more determined to handle the problem alone. God is left behind in anger and rejection. To recover, the alcoholic must allow God to become a part of life again.

Sam felt that someone had told the leader about him and that he was saying all this because it was his first day in this meditation group. He realized that, as his problem had progressed, he had made the God he knew from his days at the Baptist church less and less powerful. His life had been a progress of doing more and depending less on God or anyone. That first group helped Sam see the past twenty years from a new perspective. From that moment on, Sam knew he was in the right place. The rest of the day Sam would take the advice of the leader and meditate on the phrase "Let go and let God." He realized that in order to put his life back together, he needed to heal the spiritual wounds that had separated him from God. He could not have had a better beginning for recovery.

The next part of that morning was spent with ten other patients in a group with a counselor. Everyone introduced himself or herself to Sam and briefly told him about his or her problem. Sam was amazed that some had been addicted to Valium, some heroin, some diet pills, and some just "plain ol' alcohol out of a bottle." After the short introductions, Sam listened to a fellow patient talk about his feelings of loss and disappointment, how all of his life had come short of his expectations, and the grief he felt inside. Even though he had accumulated great wealth, life was empty and meaningless. Sam could not believe what this guy was saying. It was exactly what he had felt for years. After group, Sam asked him if he had shared those things because it was Sam's first day in group. The patient assured Sam that there would be many coincidences like that. He told him that each person was different, with a different set of circumstances, but that the commonality of a life out of control had brought them all together. Together, helping each other, they could all find the peace, happiness, meaning, and fulfillment they had wanted for so long.

The patient's prediction was true. Sam encountered many coincidences that left him feeling singled out. It happened in the lecture that morning when the presenter talked about the need to handle anger constructively. He discussed how an alcoholic grows angrier as life drifts out of control. He described the common tendency to "stuff" the anger until it becomes so intense that an episode of rage finally diffuses the emotions, but the destruction caused by the rage causes greater anger inside the alcoholic. Sam was amazed at the description of how normal, wonderful people become bitter and angry along the path of alcoholism. It described his own life perfectly. He wistfully recalled those days when he was calm and at peace with the world.

Many patients have a hard time knowing where to start to work on themselves. They expect someone to do for them what they must do for themselves. Sam was fortunate in that he knew just where to begin with his anger. From the morning session he knew he was not alone in that problem. The presentation had touched a nerve with Sam, and he was ready to begin to work on his recovery. He knew he had a problem and accepted responsibility for doing something about it. It was an important step toward recovery. From the beginning he realized that recovery would not be something that would happen to him; it would be something he would have to work toward.

The rest of Sam's day included a private session with his counselor, an afternoon of aerobics and volleyball, and a time alone to read and listen to a tape on recovery. The day ended with the patients attending a meeting of Alcoholics Anonymous. Many patients resist the treatment process in every way. They fight for the right to do it alone or do it differently. But Sam was compliant from the beginning. He was motivated to change. Nothing he had done on his own had produced change. He welcomed the help for himself and his family.

The rest of treatment consisted of more sharing in groups, and an increasing openness and honesty with the other patients. There were lectures, discussion groups, exercise sessions, and time alone to read, listen, and reflect. A process was taking place within Sam that involved the program material, the staff, and the other patients. Everyone struggling together in the process of recovery ushered Sam into the sixth and most desirable personality of the alcoholic, the sober one.

The longer Sam's recovery continued, the higher the quality of his sobriety became. The quality of life improved for the other family members also. The entire family participated in the family program at the treatment center. They followed it up with weekly aftercare meetings at the hospital. Everyone in the family attended some type of self-help or recovery support group. Recovery became a family project. Within six months of Sam's admittance to treatment, he began to feel more comfortable as a nondrinker than he ever had as a drinker, and the family started to feel comfortable with Sam's new role as a sober father. Sam and his family were experiencing something available to all alcoholics but experienced by too few: sobriety.

In those initial days of Sam's sobriety, he began to emerge out of his misery and into a manageable life-style. His expectations of others became more realistic, as did his expectations of himself. He was no longer deluged with extreme guilt over the past or paralyzing anxiety of the future. He was able to deal with the present. He spent his time on the "here and now" rather than the "there and never." Sam was rooted in *today*, and he could handle that. He could be comfortable with himself and others just relaxing. His mind no longer raced out of control. Serenity was something that Sam enjoyed for the first time in his life. One-day-at-a-time living suited him just fine.

Sam began to deal with reality on a daily basis. He stopped lying and settled for all that the truth had to offer. With the truth he destroyed his own illusions to produce a world that was real—full of feelings, communication, and growth. His work was not free of problems, but they were manageable. Sam handled the problems of the real world by sharing the load with those around him. He dealt with what he could and left the rest for some other day or someone else. He accepted his limitations and inability to change the entire world. He had made a 180-degree turn in his life. The change was obvious to everyone who knew him.

In the process of dealing with reality in the present, Sam began to develop a calmness that was noticeable to his family and friends. Because of the manageability of life and his new perspective, the emotional extremes he had experienced for so long were no longer necessary. Rather than avoiding Sam, people wanted to be around him. He had something that others wanted to share. A predictable inner support gave him security and the courage to triumph one more day. The consequences of drinking were no longer producing daily disasters, and Sam Jorgenson was making peace with the world. His selfish attitudes changed into genuine care and concern for others. The remarkable reversal amazed and pleased many friends and acquaintances. They liked what they saw in the new Sam Jorgenson.

While drinking and even after he had stopped, Sam had felt

an emptiness inside that gnawed at him as he sank into the swamp of worthlessness. Life had no meaning, and he felt nothing but discontent. Now, in the state of sobriety, he was beginning to develop a sense of purpose. He knew that life was more than just a daily battle for personal survival. He felt good about himself, about what he was doing and the direction his life was taking. Once freed from his prison of addiction, he was able to invest his best in his family, friends, and employees. His life had meaning, and he felt he had a reason to live. Nothing gave his life more meaning than when he shared his experience with fellow strugglers. He was motivated to help others experience the freedom he felt through sobriety. His attitude changed so radically that he felt that if his misery could prevent someone else from going through what he had, then it was all worth it. He filled the void with new hope for life, which he shared with others.

As Sam's drinking had progressed to more destructive stages, he had experienced a growing discomfort with everything and everyone around him. With the powers of addiction and withdrawal stretching his limits to tolerate massive internal and external irritations, his discomfort had become intense. But now he was learning to find his own comfort, no matter how uncomfortable the situation or people surrounding him might be. He did not expect the world to meet his demands and no longer acted as if it should revolve around him. His destructive perfectionist attitudes were replaced by healthy acceptance. His focus shifted from what was not perfect to locating that which was okay. As he allowed others their own imperfections, it became easier to accept and manage his own. It had been years since he had been able to love and accept people just the way they are. In his sobriety, his perspective was different on how to live and let live. It was a perspective that provided him and those around him with comfort rather than irritation.

Lastly, but most important, a spiritual perspective of life grew out of Sam's sobriety. As a young man in the Baptist church, he had known there was a spiritual dimension to life. His drinking completely destroyed it. He had been through a lot since his church days. He had become alienated from anything and anyone who was affiliated with church, religion, or God. Sam would beg for God to help him, then moments later proclaim that there was no God. He had doubted God's existence as the alcohol had become more powerful. It was his guilt and shame that had separated him from God. Now it was his ability to forgive himself that was freeing him to consider God as a power greater than himself. As he accepted God's forgiveness for himself, he was able to accept God's forgiveness for others. After a long journey through spiritual barrenness, he finally felt connected to those around him and to God.

Recovering alcoholics have many different concepts of God. Some understand God as a power greater than themselves, experienced through the care and concern of the members of a self-help group. Some go years without a belief in God. They have been so separated for so long that it takes years to heal the spiritual wounds. But in Sam's sobriety, God as he understood Him was the God of the Bible, and it was on that understanding that his spiritual life was founded. Whatever the foundation, spiritual recovery is essential for sobriety that fosters a richly satisfying life-style. It starts with a search for truth and purpose. For most it results in the discovery of God, the Creator.

In growing spiritually, Sam had to deal with three very important concepts. They were the keys to his own development, not only spiritually but mentally and socially as well. Those keys opened a way to maturity that could come in no other manner. Those three concepts were responsibility, commitment, and discipline. The three words, welded together in a plan for development, launched Sam into the realm of genuine spirituality. Spirituality is sometimes misunderstood as something spooky or mystical, but when approached from these three concepts, it is easy to understand and develop. As Sam accepted responsibility for his actions, as he disciplined his mind and body, and as he became dependable in his commitment, the spiritual fibers of his life wove an interlocking foundation on which Sam established a life that meant more than he could have ever imagined.

Sam discovered many things in his first months of recovery. The most important was that recovery takes time. It does not happen overnight. It occurs over periods of struggle, setback, and even relapse. Sam had many discouraging days, with frustrations that plunged him into unhealthy doubt. But he survived because he was involved with other human beings. When the problems were too great to be handled alone, he had people and relationships to turn to rather than a chemical in a bottle. The relationships provided enough support to keep him sober until the initial adjustments of recovery were made. With time, those supportive people, and trust in God, Sam lived a sober life. And he motivated many others to obtain sobriety also.

Sobriety, as Sam discovered, is not a state of mind free of problems or difficulties. It is not some elusive condition experienced in some distorted world of unreality. It is merely a way of life that enables a person to grow and mature as problems arise. Sobriety contrasts with the typical life-style of escape and regression in destructive alcoholic drinking. Sobriety is a struggle, entered into with a group of fellow strugglers. In the struggle there is great hope—hope for a new tomorrow and hope for a new life.

In looking back at Sam's life, the six personalities he experienced are easily identifiable. First there was the *abstainer*, that time before Sam took his first drink. He was naïve, and young and full of potential, and also of all the natural apprehensions of adolescence. Sam was pressured to drink, but he delayed the decision to do so until college.

The second state or personality was the *drinker*. In this stage, Sam's initial drinking was a positive experience. He felt as if he belonged when he drank. His drinking did not produce wild drunkenness, and he was in more control of his actions than most of his drinking friends. But the drinker changed. Like other alcoholics, Sam's tolerance increased, and so did the unpredictability of his drinking. Eventually he was able to drink so much that his body became dependent on the alcohol. It actually began to function better with alcohol in it than without it. When Sam stopped drinking, he entered into the third personality state.

The third personality was the state of *withdrawing*. As the cells craved the chemical alcohol, Sam's agitation intensified. He was irritable and obsessed with his own discomfort. He was depressed and expected those around him to cater to his need to feel normal. He became a tyrant to family and friends as each cell demanded to be replenished with alcohol. Once adapted to the chemical, his body thrived on it. Without it, his body produced misery for him and those near him.

The fourth personality was the state of *toxicity*. The more Sam drank, the more cluttered his brain became from the toxic chemicals that could not be eliminated from the body because of the great amounts being consumed. The functions of Sam's mind became greatly distorted. His thinking, memory, emotions, judgment, and willpower were greatly altered. At times he appeared mentally ill, either manic-depressive or schizophrenic. In this fourth personality state, he was beyond making rational decisions to help himself. The real person of worth and value was submerged beneath the results of withdrawal and toxicity.

The fifth personality was perhaps the most painful of all, that of the *dry* alcoholic. At last stopping the drinking and hoping to find relief, Sam only found his dilemma worsened. He was in a state of obsession, and he was miserable. Every day became a struggle to stay in control as control became more and more difficult. Finally, after a drinking episode, Sam entered treatment and began the daily process of developing the sixth personality.

The sixth and most desirable personality for Sam was the *sober* one. In sobriety Sam began to deal with the reality of today with a sense of purpose and spiritual perspective. He no longer struggled alone—he struggled in relationships with his family, friends, fellow workers, and the support of a self-help group. In his sobriety he moved from a world of defeat and despair into a world of victory and hope.

What happened to Sam has happened to thousands of others who have battled alcoholism. It is a predictable progression of problems with an established source of recovery. But for that recovery to begin, the alcoholic must be willing to do whatever it takes to stop drinking and start living. It takes courage for the alcoholic to cut away that chemical offering certain death and choose life to the fullest. Every alcoholic must come to the point Sam Jorgenson did, where he or she is willing to do whatever it takes to live. That point is like a rebirth. Certainly an old and miserable person starts to die.

CHAPTER TEN

TO BEGIN AGAIN

Alcoholism and drug addiction are devastating to individuals, families, and society at large. Nothing can destroy so many people as addiction. Once it takes hold, it eventually grabs and strangles every part of a person. But there is one wonderful characteristic about addiction that separates it from other chronic, fatal diseases: the ability of those who have it to begin again. After years, even decades, of drinking or using drugs, it is still not too late. Every addict has the ability to start over. With addiction comes the blessing of a second chance.

HITTING BOTTOM

Before a person starts over, he or she must hit bottom. Hitting bottom is the point at which recovery begins. At the bottom, a person stops manipulating, conniving, and struggling and instead, surrenders and allows others to help. When bottom is hit, denial is shattered, and the addict is able to see the evidence and the reality of the addiction process. The alcoholic's or the addict's own false hope ends, and true hope for a better life begins.

A person can hit bottom four different ways. Each one is as effective as the others in initiating recovery. The only difference is that there is an order of preference for the four methods, from least desirable to most desirable. Each one is painful, but none as painful as continuing to die in the addiction process.

The first way of hitting bottom is to lose everything. This is how most people define hitting bottom. But it is *never* necessary for an alcoholic or addict to reach this point before beginning again. Money, family, job, and self-esteem dissolve. It is by far the most painful way for a person to reach bottom. Skid rows are full of those who have progressed through years of addiction, fought to hold on to life and freedom to drink and take drugs and eventually lost it all.

When someone hits bottom by losing everything, there is very little hope for change. Of course, anyone on skid row could get sober today, and some do. Plenty of resources are available for them. The reason so few people move from this point is that the motivation to change is so low. Without a family, there is no motivation to go home again; there is no home. Without a job, there is no motivation to continue to make money. There is nothing to return to except a world that produces feelings of inferiority.

The second way people hit bottom is through a tragedy. Unlike the first method, where everything is gone, this one involves the loss of something valuable. That could be freedom, a spouse, an arm or a leg, or a child. Hospitals are full of cancer and cardiac patients who plead to God for survival. They try to persuade God to help them through the crisis. They bargain that they will be good, go to church, and a lot of other things that do not happen once the crisis subsides. Alcoholics and drug addicts are the same way. Only, when they really hit bottom, they make a change forever.

It is sad that so many alcoholics and addicts hit bottom by losing something valuable. Many lives, limbs, and jobs are needlessly wasted before the person declares that enough has been lost. At that point the addicts' recovery can begin. But this usually occurs after wasted years of drinking and drug use.

The third means of hitting bottom is through intervention. Friends, family, employer, and significant others gather to precipitate a crisis for the addict, a controlled event in which the alcoholic is forced to face the reality of addiction. In a planned setting, each person close to the addict tells of the events that have happened as consequences of drinking and using drugs. The person tells how he or she felt when it happened, then strongly recommends that the person obtain help. The emotional power and force of this type of confrontation usually is enough to motivate the person to seek help. It allows the addict to hit bottom in a controlled setting. All is not lost, and no tragedy need precede it. All that is needed is for those close to the alcoholic to care enough to confront.

The alcoholic does not have to wait for people to intervene before hitting bottom but can initiate the fourth form of hitting bottom at any time. The fourth method is the most desirable. It is simply making the decision to change. It is the ability to say, "Enough is enough. It is time to change and try a new way to live." As Alcoholics Anonymous puts it, "I'm sick and tired of being sick and tired." Hitting bottom by making a decision requires brutal honesty. The addict must accept reality before friends or a tragedy force such an acceptance. When the alcoholic or addict finally decides to get well, there is no need for further hurt or harm. The new beginning is the new reality.

Anyone can remain the same. Anyone can wallow in self-pity and misery. It takes no courage to justify your situation or blame someone for being there, but it takes great courage to change a situation. The brave finally refuse to remain a victim of heredity, past decisions, or mistreatment from others. They finally decide that there is no need to let only the rest of the world enjoy life. Life and its pleasures are available to all, even alcoholics and drug addicts, if they are willing to break out of the chains of addiction and into the freedom of recovery.

Much of the material in this book deals with the disease concept of alcoholism. The case has been stated for a genetic predisposition that leads to addiction, which leads to focusing not on the guilt of the past but on recovery in the future. But I must restate an important point: *it does not matter what causes alcoholism or drug addiction.* Whether it is genetic or environmental, if you have it, you are the only one who can do something about it. You must accept responsibility for changing your life. No one can do it for you. Some may try, but no one will.

From time to time, I have counseled alcoholics and addicts who have been brought into the office kicking and screaming by a spouse. As we discussed the need for treatment, the addict or alcoholic resistant to treatment would often say something like "It is not that bad yet!" This ridiculous statement is a defense that has kept too many people from accepting the need to obtain help. I have encouraged those people to participate in an exercise that I invite you to try. If you have an alcohol or a drug problem but do not think it is bad enough to require help, this may help you see the need to act now and the futility of waiting.

Take a piece of paper and a pencil. Write at the top HOW BAD IT HAS TO GET. Next write down, one by one, circumstances that would indicate a need to seek treatment. Cover each area of your life to figure out at what point in the progression you would finally reach out and seek help. Would your husband or wife have to leave you? Would you have to cough up blood? Would you have to lose your job? Would you have to have cirrhosis of the liver? Would you have to lose control and really embarrass yourself in public? Would you have to beat your spouse to see the need to start over? Would you have to end up in jail for drunk driving? Or would it take killing a child while driving under the influence? If you honestly try to list just what it is you are waiting for, you may come to see that there is absolutely no need to wait. Please don't.

There are also those who are not alcoholic or addicted but are trapped by a spouse's chemical use. They, too, must ask: "How bad does it have to get?" How much worse does the problem have to become before he or she decides to act in order to help the person who is chemically dependent? Often the wife or husband will not take action because of guilt. The drug-dependent person hooks the family into believing that *they* are wrong, that *they* have the real problem, so the "coalcoholic" refuses to act, refuses to even mention the problem. The refusal could arise from guilt, but also probably from fear of reprisal.

There are others close to the alcoholic who are willing to take action, but nothing they do or try to do seems to work, and it only makes the situation worse or more volatile. Those coalcoholics, codependents, or significant others will fail at trying to solve the problem alone. What they need to do is reach out for professional help. Specially trained counselors can help each family member learn behaviors that will motivate the alcoholic to change rather than to drink or drug even more. The help can be obtained in complete confidentiality. The sick spouse or parent need not know.

The courage to confront is often beyond the grasp of one individual. One person is rarely enough to motivate the addicted man or woman to obtain help. But when loved ones band together, the power is greater than the person or the force of addiction. The intervention process mentioned earlier can be the method that will change the course of addiction for the whole family. The courage to confront ought to be replaced with the courage to call an intervention counselor to discuss the situation. Intervention can help the alcoholic or addict hit bottom and so, for the first time in years, reach for the top.

It is important to remember why some people cannot make

a positive decision to change. First, they are living in a delusional world full of denial and rationalization. These defense mechanisms have become vital survival tools; it is almost impossible to give them up. They have served the alcoholic or addict well. Second, the chemical both distorts reality and produces sick minds. It is unrealistic to believe that an irrational person with a sick mind is going to make a rational decision to get well. Without some form of intervention, it probably will not happen. People close to the alcoholic or addict must be willing to do for the person what he or she may not be able to do.

The most common excuse for not acting or intervening is the belief that the alcoholic or addict must want help before being helped. So the family sits around and watches the physical abuse, watches the job vanish, and watches the money go away. They wait until the addict becomes so sick and miserable that there is no choice but to get well. What a waste of much of life! The alcoholic and the addict want help. They may deny that fact to the bitter end, but down inside, they know that something is wrong and that it must be fixed. Intervention at first brings fear and anger, but finally a tremendous feeling of relief. The alcoholic and the addict know that the suffering will all come to an end one day. That it ends without a tragedy is a relief that the person will appreciate throughout sobriety.

There is never an easy way to help an alcoholic or an addict. There is no set pattern or plan that will work for everyone. It is always a struggle to wean someone away from the instant relief drugs offer and into the painful process of change. But those who do not give up the struggle usually reap the reward of watching a person regain self-esteem and a life of meaning and purpose.

Many different resources are available to the alcoholic or addict who decides to obtain help. It was not long ago that hospital beds and counselors and self-help groups were out of reach for the addict, but fortunately, that has changed. A community might be missing some components of treatment, but they are probably not too far away. Traveling to obtain help should not stand in the way. It is common to drive for miles or fly across the country to seek the best cancer or cardiac care; it should be no less a priority for the addict. Addiction is just as deadly as cancer and heart disease.

Treatment resources vary in length of time and cost of treatment. They also vary in philosophy. There are some key factors to consider when looking at a treatment resource to ensure that it will provide high-quality care. I will go into these in discussing the categories of these resources. Within each category may be found both helpful groups and possibly harmful resources, but from working with treatment centers for almost a decade, I have found most to be staffed with capable counselors and other professionals who are dedicated completely to helping alcoholics or addicts. Rather than waiting to compare the quality or perceived quality of a resource, it is far better to act and utilize something than to allow the addiction process to go on. The following are some of the resources that are available.

SELF-HELP GROUPS

The self-help movement has been a revolutionary development for alcoholics and addicts. While other resources were nonexistent, the self-help groups filled a tremendous void and provided help when it was otherwise unavailable. The early self-help groups provided something else extremely important, the proof that the addict and alcoholic *can* get well. They were the first to show that an alcoholic need not go crazy or die. Because of them, an alternative was available.

Today it seems that there is an overabundance of "anonymous" groups and support groups. For almost every problem imaginable, there is an anonymous support group that helps people deal with recovery from that problem—overweight, gambling, debt, sexual excess. There is a reason for the proliferation of those groups—they work. They help real people with real problems. They are based on the principles established by Alcoholics Anonymous. Those principles are available to help anyone who has a desire to stop drinking or engaging in other compulsive, destructive behavior. Alcoholics Anonymous, the first real source of help for alcoholics, is also the most effective means by which people stay sober.

Self-help groups and Alcoholics Anonymous are full of people who have something in common. They have reached a point with their problem where they have been able to say, "I cannot handle this alone." They call upon the strength and support of the group to help them do what they realize cannot be done alone. Within the group there is a common bond of fellow strugglers who have followed the same path through addiction. For those who have felt alienation and isolation, the self-help group is a place to feel wanted. No one is rejected there.

The value of not feeling alone is a very important dimension to self-help and anonymous groups and can make involvement in them attractive. There is another dimension that is much more vital to long-term sobriety: accountability. Within the group there is a special source of accountability, because everyone in the group has "been there." The alcoholic cannot play games, deny, or rationalize, because those in the group who have been there can see through the connivings and the bull. That type of accountability forces the alcoholic to be honest. When the games stop, real recovery can begin.

The truly valuable self-help groups are not just sources of fellowship and accountability but also provide steps toward spiritual growth and maturity. Through the support of the group and by allowing God to take care of the unchangeable, the alcoholic can follow steps that allow for spiritual growth and development that had been stifled by addiction. Those steps include elements such as confession, restitution, and carrying the message to other people who are addicted. When the steps and the program are adopted, the individual overcomes the maturity deficit incurred by alcoholism or addiction. Concepts like responsibility, delayed gratification, and discipline become a way of life.

Here are twelve steps of Alcoholics Anonymous, which are in essence also the foundation of many other recovery programs:

1. We admitted that we were powerless over alcohol—that our lives had become unmanageable.
2. Came to believe that a Power greater than ourselves could restore us to sanity.
3. Made a decision to turn our will and our lives over to the care of God *as we understood Him.*
4. Made a searching and fearless moral inventory of ourselves.
5. Admitted to God, to ourselves, and to another human being the exact nature of our wrongs.
6. Were entirely ready to have God remove all these defects of character.
7. Humbly asked Him to remove our shortcomings.

8. Made a list of all persons we had harmed, and became willing to make amends to them all.

9. Made direct amends to such people whenever possible, except when to do so would injure them or others.

10. Continued to take personal inventory, and when we were wrong, promptly admitted it.

11. Sought through meditation and prayer to improve our conscious contact with God *as we understood Him*, praying only for knowledge of His will and the power to carry that out.

12. Having had a spiritual awakening as a result of these steps, we tried to carry this message to alcoholics and to practice these principles in all our affairs.

To those who want it, self-help groups provide a lot of help and support in recovery. There really is one for everyone. None are better or more effective than Alcoholics Anonymous or Narcotics Anonymous. Some groups serve the very special needs of certain groups and professions. There are groups that meet that are composed only of airline pilots; others are for physicians. Some groups meet specific religious needs; there are Christian AA groups that address the higher power specifically as Jesus Christ. If an alcoholic finds one group a bit uncomfortable, there is always another that will suit him or her better. It is merely a matter of determination and searching.

The fact that the AA and self-help groups are voluntary makes them attractive to many, but it presents a problem to those looking for any excuse to return to the drug of their choice. They choose to try the group once, but if everything is not just perfect, they may not choose to go back for years. I have often encountered people in treatment who say that AA did not work for them, that they tried it years ago and it was not helpful. Only when they enter a formal program that requires them to go to a certain number of meetings do they experience the hope to be found in the fellowship of Alcoholics Anonymous. AA in conjunction with a formal treatment program can be highly effective, because the alcoholic is forced to "shut up and listen" long enough to grasp the value of the group.

In my opinion, every alcoholic should attend Alcoholics Anonymous, and every drug addict should attend either Alcoholics Anonymous or Narcotics Anonymous. To me, anyone who refuses to go is not totally committed to staying sober. Too many people have become well through those groups for there to be any reason for refusing to attend. It is as if a cancer patient, terminally ill, were to refuse an injection that has helped more people recover than any other treatment. No responsible program or treatment is going to provide long-term help for the alcoholic or addict unless attendance in AA or NA is strongly encouraged. I would never refer someone to a program that did not stress the value and importance of Alcoholics Anonymous or Narcotics Anonymous. When other programs have disbanded or moved or gone out of business, AA and NA will still be there!

INPATIENT TREATMENT

It seems that you cannot watch television for very long without seeing a commercial for a privately funded program or a public program housed in a hospital for the treatment of alcoholism or drug addiction. For the past twelve years, empty hospital beds have been used for addiction recovery through these inpatient treatment programs. Now more than ever, there is stiff competition among those centers to attract patients. Such programs often come under criticism by those who distrust their profit motive and may question the cost or length of stay or treatment methods. The visibility of the programs certainly makes them open targets, but a closer look reveals what is at the heart of this industry geared to help those with alcohol and drug problems.

I should say first that my opinions about inpatient treatment are admittedly biased. I have been associated with inpatient treatment in some way ever since my college days. My belief in their value and worth comes from experience as counselor, program director, and executive of two companies that managed inpatient programs. The experience has provided me with the proof that these programs are a wonderful addition to society; I have seen at first hand the thousands who have been helped through them. Before carping, the critics should talk to those who recaptured their lives through these great institutions.

There is a simple way to evaluate programs. If someone must have assurance before using the services of a hospital-based program, it is not hard to obtain. No matter what organization or corporation heads up the program, its effectiveness is measured unit by unit and facility by facility. First, one should talk to the staff who work there. If the staff are well trained, composed of both recovering and nonrecovering counselors, that is a good sign; such a combination of staff is known to increase effectiveness. (By "nonrecovering," I mean, of course, someone who has never been an alcoholic or an addict, not one who is still caught in the addiction!) The recovering team members provide a dimension of credibility and trust for the early patient because they have "been through it." Early on, they can often establish fast rapport with someone who is still not completely convinced of the need to get sober. Nonrecovering people are also an asset by providing objectivity. A recovering person may believe that all addicts need to do exactly as he or she did to get well, but the nonrecovering person may be more open and flexible in looking at components of a recovery plan. Both recovering and nonrecovering people have a place in treatment. Both should be trained to skillfully manage and treat alcoholics, addicts, and their families.

There is something even more important than top-notch training in counselors: the dimension of caring. Of course, no one can teach another person to care; you cannot quantitatively measure the caring factor. When you observe a group of caring, concerned professionals, their desire to help becomes obvious. It is important to know that rigidity and insensitivity are not part of the treatment process. Every new patient and family member should be treated as a unique individual with unique concerns. If that understanding is not found in the program's staff, it is probably not the best program.

The staff *are* the program. The quality is determined by their competence in the treatment process, and their competence can be measured only by the results that they produce. This can best be determined by talking to ex-patients and graduates of the program. For real insight into the program, ask the staff to allow you to talk to an ex-patient. Ask the person what it was like and how well he or she was treated. Ask about quality of life after drinking. Is the person merely off the alcohol for a while, or has there been a radical life-style change? Be sure and ask about the individual's family and how well the team dealt with them. If you find that the graduates of the program are well adjusted and into secure recovery, and that its team is a caring and competent one, the program is probably of excellent quality.

Some very important elements of inpatient treatment programs foster the maximum potential for recovery. These elements are medical detoxification, active treatment, family involvement, and aftercare. Let's look at each one of these elements briefly.

Medical Detoxification

This is one of the greatest benefits of inpatient treatment. A lot can go wrong, and often does, in the early withdrawal stages. It is best to go through withdrawal under the care of competent nurses and physicians who can bring the alcohol or drug levels in the system down in a controlled fashion. When this is accomplished properly, the addict or alcoholic remains in treatment. When it is mismanaged, the need for a drink or medication drives the person to leave and seek some form of self-medication. The best security for a new start is a well-managed detoxification regimen. When correctly supervised, it allows the alcoholic or addict to slip comfortably out of the addictive power of the chemical and into the positive reinforcements for recovery.

Active Treatment Phase

When detoxification is over, active treatment can begin. It is in this phase that the five aspects of recovery are addressed. No aspect is to be left out—they are all equally important. Here is what should be covered at a minimum in each area:

Physical
- How to relax
- How to eat to maintain a stable blood sugar level
- How to exercise and tone the body

Mental
- Information on addiction and how it affects the individual and the family
- Lectures on a new way of thinking positively to achieve success
- Tapes on how to live more effectively
- Speakers who have been through addiction and recovery

Emotional
- Group counseling to process guilt, fear, anger
- Individual counseling to meet specific emotional needs and problems

- Open discussion of thoughts, ideas, and feelings about the past, present, and future

Social

- Plans on new places to go and new things to do
- Assistance in eliminating negative social influences
- Help in developing new positive reinforcements
- Plans to mend and develop old relationships

Spiritual

- Assistance in developing purpose and meaning in life
- Exploration of truth
- Discussions on beliefs about God and the power available through God
- Development of discipline, responsibility, and maturity

Each of these areas should be thoroughly addressed while the patient is in treatment. Whether treatment is ten days or thirty days long, it is still a short length of time to change all five dimensions of a person's life. So treatment cannot be viewed as an all-inclusive package that heals people from head to toe; it is only a place to start. While in the active treatment phase, the most valuable accomplishment is not resolution of problems but the development of long-term plans that will one day allow the patient to resolve the problems. If a person in treatment is not making post-treatment plans, then treatment is a waste of time.

Some programs include aversion therapy in the active treatment phase. It should never be mandatory but can be a useful option for treatment. Aversion to alcohol helps a person "buy some time." A lot of people do not recover because they are unable to go without alcohol long enough to establish a solid recovery program, and such people have been helped by this method. Though controversial, it can be a valuable adjunct to treatment if managed by competent professionals in a caring way.

The active treatment phase is a launching pad for the voyage toward a new life. It forms the foundation for the recovery program. It allows sobriety to begin in a safe, supportive environment. Perhaps the most valuable aspect of the active treatment phase is the interaction with other patients. Seeing, knowing, talking with others who have been down into the addiction valley and are climbing up the other side is immensely helpful in breaking out of isolation and alienation. Most of what happens in a program happens between the patients and residents. The staff are there to facilitate that interaction. The only reason a person would not benefit from it is lack of participation. No staff member can force a person to be open and honest with others, but when a person risks being open and honest, recovery can begin.

Family Involvement

If the alcoholic or the addict changes but the family does not, one of two things will happen: the alcoholic or addict will relapse, or the family will break up. No program should exist without family involvement. If a person must be in treatment away from home, the treatment team should make provisions for the family to receive help locally. The best situation allows for the family to be involved in the same program with the patient. That might require renting a hotel room or finding help with child care. No barrier should be too great to prevent involvement of the family. Any program that does not address this need is inadequate.

Family issues are not resolved quickly. Some families experience extreme problems such as incest or physical abuse. Attending a couple of lectures will not mend these deep emotional scars. The family should be assisted in obtaining help after treatment is over. Many alcoholics and addicts have stayed in recovery because of a family that did not shy away from commitment to change along with the addict or alcoholic. Another important resource for long-term commitment to change is Alanon. Alanon is designed for the family and can be a tremendous support for recovery. When no other form of family treatment is affordable, Alanon is always available. It should not be considered a last resort. Just as the alcoholic should go to AA to insure long-term sobriety, every family should attend Alanon to ensure its own long-term recovery. Alanon is patterned on AA, but it should be understood that its purpose is to help the families heal themselves, not train them as therapists for the alcoholic. The alcoholic's recovery and the family's recovery are linked, but the success of one does not depend on the other.

Aftercare

Aftercare provides valuable support during the transition from inpatient treatment back to the real world. It is also a tremendous support for life, especially when the alcoholic or addict is feeling more obsessed with the idea of drinking or using drugs. Aftercare consists of group sessions whereby the therapy that began in treatment can continue through total recovery. Aftercare should be a service included in the total package of inpatient treatment and not be an extra charge.

Aftercare is such an important element of treatment that it should not be left to amateurs. Professional counselors should handle the groups, because they can be volatile. People return to the groups after facing the reality of job stress, family pressure, and lack of social support. The person who in treatment thought sobriety would be easy comes to aftercare with deep problems concerning the reality of just how tough it is to go one day without a drink or a drug. A professional counselor or a recovering person with years of sobriety needs to be involved in resolving these issues with the ex-patients. A program that ends treatment on the last day of an inpatient stay is not providing adequate support during the difficult periods of initial sobriety. If aftercare is not a priority for the center, there is a good chance that the directors of that program are interested in something other than quality.

Inpatient treatment is a wonderful resource for recovery. It allows the family and the addict to be a part of the process, to regroup and develop objectivity about the problem and the future. Most provide a safe environment in which an addict or alcoholic can begin the recovery process. The two greatest assets of these centers are the people who staff them and the people who are there to be helped. The combination of a caring staff and support of fellow patients can be just the right mix for a solid foundation of recovery. If money or insurance is available to pay for these programs, quick progress can be made through their treatment. Because of their success, thousands have tasted the sweetness of sobriety.

THE HALFWAY HOUSE

The halfway house is a place where people can go off to work during the day and return in the evening to an environment supportive of recovery. During the evening, residents usually hear lectures, see films, conduct their own Alcoholics Anonymous or Narcotics Anonymous meetings, or go out as a group to AA or NA meetings nearby. In some areas the halfway house is a run-down, shabby little house that people avoid passing; in others it is a luxurious home where physicians and attorneys feel comfortable while getting their lives back together. Because of the supportive environment, the evening sessions, and the strong emphasis on AA and NA, the halfway house can be the ideal place to start recovery. It is also valuable when family problems make the home unbearable; the recovering person can move into a halfway house while the family is undergoing treatment. When the more volatile emotional issues are resolved, the addict or alcoholic can move back home again.

In most halfway houses, the residents learn to live responsibly and with others. Everyone pitches in to cook, clean up, and handle the everyday maintenance of the place. Anyone not willing to help with the chores is confronted about selfishness and ego. It is very valuable training in learning to consider others before self. Halfway houses are great places. They cost very little and are usually staffed with very caring people. If a community wanted to make a vital contribution to help alcoholics and addicts, it would build or develop more halfway houses, some for men, some for women, and some for adolescents. The availability of this type of resource, affordable and located within the community, can be a crucial element in a community plan to fight alcohol and drug problems.

OUTPATIENT TREATMENT

Outpatient treatment allows a person to work, live at home, and at the same time receive help in working on sobriety. Most of the programs meet two to four evenings a week, with some daytime sessions for evening and night workers. Programs consist of lectures, films, tapes, group therapy, family therapy, and attendance at AA or NA. The quality varies, due to the organizational difficulties with the programs. Some are excellent, but others fail to provide the needed structure for the alcoholic or addict. In poorly organized programs, the dropout rate can be extremely high. If quick follow-up is not done with each patient when there is an unexplained absence, program completion becomes doubtful. Since the patient does not live on the program premises, there are thousands of reasons not to return. Effective outpatient programs take this problem into account and set up systems to ensure maximum attendance.

The other major difficulty with outpatient programs stems

from the fact that the patient is living at home. While adjusting to a life free of chemicals, the addict or alcoholic can be very difficult to live with. A family with unresolved guilt, fear, and anger can make a difficult situation even worse. The program must address this problem. Family involvement must be an internal part of the program. When the evening session breaks up, the counselor must ensure that family tensions have been lessened by the session, not intensified to an unbearable level. When sensitive to family pressure, organized to meet the need for structure of the newly recovering person, and consistently following up potential dropouts, the outpatient route can be an excellent way of starting the recovery process.

DAY TREATMENT

Day treatment is more rare than outpatient or inpatient care. It can be described in one of two ways: some call it an intensified day-long outpatient program. Others describe it as inpatient treatment with the person going home every night. Where they exist, these programs have been very successful due to their low cost and high-intensity programming. There does remain the issue of living with the family when the first days of recovery are so tense. Some industries have established day treatment programs to lower the cost of treating a great number of employees. A day treatment facility is an excellent resource, but very rare and difficult to find. It should contain all the elements of inpatient treatment except for the beds and the medical detoxification program. Like inpatient programs, its effectiveness should be measured by the quality of its staff and the sobriety of its graduates.

MULTIFAMILY GROUP THERAPY

The most exciting recent development in recovery resources is the multifamily group treatment process. They are even more rare than day treatment programs, but they produce dramatic results in the most difficult of cases. When a person enters this type of treatment, there is a very good chance of getting well; the success rate is extremely high.

What makes these programs so effective? Commitment. You cannot enter one of these programs unless both the addict or alcoholic and the family are committed to receive treatment, which means following the directives of the program. This entails *no one* in the family drinking or using drugs, weekly attendance at all meetings, and a radical change in life-style. The program combines whatever other components and resources are needed to provide comprehensive treatment for the entire family. The one who is chemically dependent might be asked to go to inpatient treatment, or a family member might be asked to see a psychiatrist. The attitude of the best of these programs is "whatever it takes."

The chemically dependent person will attend groups with other alcoholics and addicts, and he or she and the family will have family sessions with a primary counselor. There will also be large group sessions with several families. This is accompanied by individual one-to-one counseling sessions as needed. The groups go out to attend lectures on recovery together; they go to AA, NA, and Alanon meetings; they become completely committed and involved in the total recovery, in every dimension, of both the alcoholic or addict and the family.

These programs, because of their intensity, are quite expensive. It takes considerable organization and a qualified staff to run a high-quality operation and produce such an outstanding success rate. I have seen absolutely hopeless cases make a complete turnaround through involvement in a multifamily group treatment program. Though costly and time-consuming, requiring tremendous commitment, the healing of an individual and a family is very much worth it.

COUNSELORS

There are many counselors—psychologists, social workers, and a variety of other therapists—who are able to help alcoholics and addicts recover. The most effective will tell you of their limitations when the counseling begins. A counselor alone is not an acceptable method of obtaining sobriety; the counselor must be willing to refer the patient to other resources, such as inpatient or outpatient treatment, when needed. Effective counseling will be accompanied by attendance at lectures to gather additional information about the problem and recovery from it. The competent counselor will also demand attendance at Alcoholics Anonymous or Narcotics Anonymous. Nor will the effective counselor forget the needs of the family, ensuring that they, too, are receiving help.

It is all too rare that a counselor will know how to work with alcoholics and addicts. He or she will often try to find out why a person drinks or uses drugs rather than develop a strategy for not using alcohol or drugs, one day at a time. Many counselors will never even approach the alcohol or drug problem, considering it secondary to deeper-rooted issues. Although this is comfortable for the alcoholic or addict, it is destructive and prevents the person from finding the way to recovery without chemicals. Before a life is turned over to a counselor, therapist, or psychiatrist for guidance, it is important to be sure that the person is trained and experienced in chemical dependency. Especially must it be established that the counselor understands that total abstinence is the only way to maintain a valuable lifestyle. When counselors are trained, competent, and experienced, they can provide an excellent means of beginning again.

1-800-227-LIFE

It is hard to know where to turn when seeking help for drug and alcohol problems. If resources are available, it is hard to evaluate whether or not any one resource is solid, credible, and reputable. It is for these reasons that 1-800-227-LIFE was established. No matter what you are hooked on, the people who handle the phones at 1-800-227-LIFE will help you find the best resource for your problem. Many thousands of people have called and been directed toward recovery through a local resource. The people who handle the phones have been thoroughly trained to help people find the best resource. 1-800-227-LIFE is a safe, easy place to start over. All information remains completely confidential. Calling can be a first step toward a new life of purpose and meaning.

The bad news is that alcoholism and drug addiction is a terrible problem affecting millions of lives. The good news is that there are many resources available to help those affected by the problem. Where there was a void fifty years ago, there are now wonderful programs that lead people into recovery and out of deadly addiction. There is no excuse for a person not recovering from alcoholism or drug addiction—no excuse except an unwillingness to do whatever it takes. When the point is reached that an alcoholic or addict is finally ready to do whatever it takes, the resources and help are waiting. The following chapter explores the process for which these resources and help exist: recovery.

CHAPTER ELEVEN

RECOVERY

The process of recovery is approached by various professionals, trained in distinct disciplines, from many different angles. The positive thinker believes that recovery can come from a new attitude. The nutritionist might advocate a strict diet, free of sugar and processed foods, as *the* way to beat addiction. A sociologist might dwell on the need for a complete change of environment. The minister may demand instant conversion as a means to achieve sobriety, while the psychologist believes that the key to recovery is the resolution of personal conflict and emotional trauma. Each professional tends to focus on his or her area of personal training and expertise. The result of these disparate approaches is often something other than recovery. Instead of entering recovery, the alcoholic or addict ends up on a tangent that produces temporary results and an unbalanced life-style.

It is important to recognize that none of the preceding approaches is bad or destructive. In fact, each one is very helpful to the person trying to overcome the devastation of alcohol or drugs. But recovery must encompass every area of a person's life, not just the alcoholic or addict, but every family member. When this occurs, sobriety and recovery become meaningful foundations of a new way of life.

Another hazard addicts and alcoholics encounter is those people so hung up on the cause of the problem that they do not help people search for a solution. Seeking the "why" offers little help with "what to do." Much of this book has been written in an attempt to dispel myths about the nature of alcoholism; but that information is secondary in importance to what to do to solve the problem. Millions have found answers to alcohol and drug problems, and those answers are available to anyone with the courage to seek help. Intellectual pursuit or psychological study does not move a person one step closer to recovery. Recovery comes when the intellectualization and denial end, allowing the steps toward recovery to be followed.

Note also that recovery is not the stopping of anything. Of course, the alcoholic must stop drinking and the drug addict must stop using drugs, but that is just the necessary precondition to recovery, to starting a new life. Recovery demands the willingness to change every aspect of life. Anyone who continues to drink and drug simply has not made the commitment or faced the pain needed to change. When the commitment is made, change will occur, but it is a lifetime commitment, which must be renewed every day.

Everyone travels his or her own unique road toward addiction and through it. Therefore, there is no cookie cutter approach that will stamp out a new life-style for every individual, though there are some principles that seem to apply in almost every case of meaningful sobriety. The problem with saying "almost every case" is that it implies exceptions to the principles, and everyone wants to be an exception. One of the most common statements made in treatment is "I am different!" All the same, there are some exceptions. Some people have had an instantaneous or spontaneous recovery that has changed every aspect of life, but those instances are very rare. Rather than trying to prove that one is the exception, it is better to adhere to the principles that have helped so many.

PRINCIPLE NO. 1: CONFESSION

It is human nature to cover up our problems. People do it through escape, isolation, denial, and rationalization. Most people go through life painfully continuing to cover up and hide rather than face the pain of changing. They take the path of least resistance and experience a life of extreme conflict. The key to a satisfying life is not someone's ability to mask and hide, but a willingness to open up and uncover what is beneath a sick and fragmented shell of personality.

No one recovers in secret. There must come a time in every alcoholic's or addict's life when the need to open up is faced. Hope and healing lie in openness. In hiding there is only continued misery. Every alcoholic and drug addict must be willing to say, "I have a problem"—and further, to admit that the problem is not a parent, spouse, child, or job. There must be an open admission that the problem is a chemical and that the problem can no longer be handled alone. And that confession must accompany a willingness to receive help from others.

It is difficult—it seems almost impossible—but it is the beginning of a new life. It is so simple, yet it escapes so many. The impact of making the decision can be lessened if it is done in steps. I recommend practicing with a stranger over the phone. Call a counselor who works a hot line (like 1-800-227-LIFE) and anonymously admit that you have a problem. You will find that it is not so very hard, and the ground will not shake nor lightning strike from the sky. But it will be a beginning, and it will make confession in person one step closer. It will allow openness to seem a little more possible. Once you can open up to another human being, admit the problem, and ask for help, recovery can begin.

PRINCIPLE NO. 2: LONG-TERM SUPPORT

People who recover do so with the help and support of others. The principles of openness and confession must be linked to an ever-expanding system of support. Support must transcend the initial confession process and encompass other areas. As recovery becomes more meaningful, the alcoholic must be willing to deal openly beyond the level of "I used to drink or take drugs." It must move into areas such as "Now that I do not drink, I am having problems with my children." In other words, the focus cannot remain just on past alcoholic or addicted behavior. It must encompass every aspect of life.

A person needs support in the difficult times; recovery allows that support to be rendered when needed. The alcoholic and the addict need someone to give them a pat on the back or a word of encouragement. This positive reinforcement counters the negative pressure to drink or do drugs. It allows the recovering addict or alcoholic to find a safe place in which to turn in times of trouble. Support is needed and allows the struggling alcoholic or addict to experience total acceptance.

A source of ongoing support is necessary for another reason. As human beings, we all have problems with consistency and follow-through. It is easy for us to veer off course, no matter how strong our initial motivation. Ongoing support allows each person to have a source of accountability. The group not only encourages, it points out weaknesses and flaws in the recovery process. It permits one to suggest a slight or major alteration so that sobriety can be maintained. Accountability provides the alcoholic with the opportunity to continue to grow and to realize that recovery is never over; it must be continual, a part of each day.

Many wonderful sources of ongoing long-term support are available. Certainly Alcoholics Anonymous and Narcotics Anonymous are vital to long-term sobriety. Support groups can be church groups, group therapy, recovery groups, close friends, and especially the family. As each group becomes a source of support and accountability, life becomes easier and more congruent. When the need to hide is lessened, the opportunity to be real is expanded. Without this ever-expanding network of support, recovery is guaranteed to be only temporary.

PRINCIPLE NO. 3: FAMILY INVOLVEMENT

Addicts and alcoholics need families, especially families supportive of sobriety. If an alcoholic or drug addict does not have one, it may be possible to "adopt" a "family" of supportive friends. Recovery, especially in early months and years, is a difficult proposition, and the alcoholic and addict must have as much help as possible. A difficult, negative family can throw a person into relapse if it is allowed to take control. Most people who recover do so with at least one family member who helps with the recovery process. Of course, a person *can* stay sober without a supportive family, but the process—and life itself—is so much more enjoyable when everyone works together.

Alanon is a great place to start in developing a healthy, supportive family. The family may need more than Alanon, or the family component of a treatment center program. Nothing short of intensive family therapy will bring some families back together in support of recovery. There is a lot of needless divorce and relapse because of the family's unwillingness to get help. When families see recovery as something everyone must do, there is hope for long-term sobriety and a healthy family.

The three principles of recovery combine to begin a new life for the alcoholic or addict. Openness, support, and family recovery work together to free the chemically dependent person from addiction. Unless each principle is in place, a solid base for a system of recovery can't be formed. When such a foundation is established, the recovery system can grow to balance and encompass every area of life. The five dimensions of the recovery system can form a fortress that protects the recovering person from relapse. Built on a strong foundation, they are the greatest guarantee of long-term sobriety.

DIMENSION NO. 1: PHYSICAL

The first dimension of a complete system of recovery is physical, or physiological, recovery. Physiological recovery involves both the freeing of the system from addicting chemicals and repair of body tissue damaged by drugs and alcohol. It also involves eating in such a way as to reduce mood swings and stabilize emotions. This dimension, though frequently neglected, is important to allow the healthy development of other dimensions.

Detoxification, exercise, nutrition, and relaxation combine to form the physiological component of the recovery system. When these are pursued, all the other components of recovery are easier to manage and remain more stable. Anyone interested in complete recovery must start with the body. Many people experience extreme difficulty in recovery because they have not fully developed the physiological dimension. New ease can be experienced when the body is given major priority in recovery.

Detoxification

The cleansing of the body, or the elimination of addicting chemicals from the body, is the first essential for recovery. Complete detoxification of the system is vital in developing a healthy recovery program. If detoxification is improperly handled, the recovery process is abandoned and relapse is instant. To usher the addict into recovery, detoxification controls the withdrawal from an addictive chemical by the use of lessening doses of a substance that can be easily administered and controlled. Alcohol, Valium, or Catapress are some of the substances used to control withdrawal symptoms. The purposes of using any chemical in withdrawal is to make the process predictable and safe. When it is handled properly, the addict feels safe and protected from severe withdrawal symptoms that can lead to death. Another method of detoxification is called *social detox*. This method replaces the use of chemicals with the support of counselors and recovering alcoholics. It can involve steam baths, herbal drinks, and other nonchemical methods. Whether the detoxification process is social or chemical, it must be handled by experienced individuals who can react quickly if trouble develops. If severe withdrawal symptoms can be prevented, the alcoholic or drug addict will be motivated to continue in recovery.

Freeing the body of addictive chemicals does not mean that detoxification is completely over. Further steps can be taken to rid the system of other impurities that have built up in the body over the years. There are many methods utilized to flush the body free of impurities that hamper the maximum potential for recovery. If the alcoholic or addict has for years consumed a lot of junk food, highly processed foods, and foods full of unhealthy chemicals, this further detoxification step can be very helpful to a stable recovery. Enemas, repeated saunas, hot baths, and ingestion of certain substances that cling to impurities and allow them to be flushed from the system are all means used in this further level of detoxification. The more complete the detoxification process, the better, and the more comfortable long-term sobriety can be for the recovering alcoholic or addict.

Exercise

Exercise is a key component in physiological recovery. Anyone serious about high-quality sobriety should start a physical exercise program. Its level of intensity, of course, will depend on the overall condition of the body, which can best be assessed by a physician. For almost everyone, it is appropriate to exercise daily to the point of perspiration. Working up a good sweat helps facilitate the detoxification process; it will unclog pores and allow impurities to be washed out of the system.

Exercise offers other benefits. It is the most natural form of stimulation. The stimulation it provides can boost a person out of the "blahs" of depression. When the body starts to move, the mind and emotions eventually catch up and begin to move also. Clinical studies have shown the dramatic results found in depressed people when they made the effort to walk, jog, run, or swim. They are the best alternatives to lying in bed and moping about a problem. The studies reveal that exercise can greatly help establish emotional stability. The addict or alcoholic, accustomed to getting high or experiencing a rush from an unnatural substance, can learn to experience pleasant feelings as a result of exercise. When the person goes from being hooked on drugs to the natural benefits of exercise, a destructive habit is replaced with a healthy program. And of course, one great thing about exercise is that it is free.

Exercise is also a way of managing the extreme tension and stress that can build up in early recovery. It is a natural way to relax and calm down the churning daily agitation. It is a safe and natural way to manage tension instead of letting it manage you. Rather than reach for a drink or drug, the person can learn to take a walk, jog, or swim. It can return the emotions to a manageable level when tension mounts and anger flares. Whether stimulation or relaxation is wanted, exercise can produce the desired results. It is a very inexpensive means of moving into a new mood. No recovery system is complete without it.

When developing an exercise program, the family should be considered. If the family joins in, exercise can provide a source of growing communication and family involvement. Everyone can run or walk or swim together. Even if a physically challenged person is confined to a wheelchair, he or she can participate in one of those activities. Anything that allows the family to be a family while getting in shape is a great idea. Tennis, basketball, football, softball, and any number of other team sports can provide fun for the family while improving everyone's physical and mental state. When the alcoholic stops drinking, the family members may experience added stress or tension and wonder why it would develop in the midst of the alcoholic's positive change. When exercise becomes a family affair, that tension and pressure often subside, and everyone is able to feel better. When each member is allowed to participate and be involved, family healing is prompted. If families are motivated to get well, they should find an activity that will allow each person to participate in developing a stronger body and a stronger family.

Relaxation

Relaxation techniques can also help in physiological recovery. When a person goes to the effort of scheduling a time-out period for both mind and body, recovery is enhanced. No one in recovery should become so busy that there is not enough time to reflect and relax. There must be time set aside when the calmness of relaxation and meditation is allowed to soothe the entire body and mind. The individual who wants to relax and promote complete physical healing should find a safe, quiet room in which focusing on breathing and the body is easy. There are numerous techniques to fortify the value of a quiet time out. None is more valuable or effective than scheduling ten or fifteen minutes a day for simple prayer. When time is taken to stop and reenergize and reflect on life's priorities, the benefits are experienced in every dimension of recovery. Relaxation allows the body's own healing mechanism to do the best job possible. When all the external stimuli from the outside world are shut down, the healing abilities of the body are turned on. A mind and spirit refreshed from time taken to relax can help a person maintain or regain control of body, mind, and emotions.

Nutrition

It is sad to see how few people really are attuned to the value of nutrition to a healthy recovery process. Both strength and stability will come from an abandonment of junk foods. Good, nutritious food helps the body heal and mend while countering emotional instability. Often extreme mood swings can be completely eliminated through proper diet. While the emotions remain stable and the whole person is enhanced, tissue that has been destroyed from drugs and alcohol can be replenished.

The standard American diet is very high in processed food containing an overload of fat, sugar, caffeine, preservatives, and other chemicals. The reason it is called junk food is because there is so much junk in it. The recovery diet is just the opposite from the standard American diet. It is low in fat, sugar, caffeine, chemicals, and junk foods. It is high in complex carbohydrates, whole-grain breads, vegetables, and other natural, live foods. It is also limited in animal protein. On a diet of good, natural food, rather than the common junk variety, miraculous things can happen. Blood sugar levels stabilize, mood swings decrease, frantic nervousness diminishes, and more energy is generated by the individual.

Nutrition in recovery not only involves the content of what is eaten; it also must involve how and when food is eaten. The practice of eating three large meals a day should be discarded and replaced with three smaller meals and three small snacks throughout the day. This approach to food consumption can be verified as effective by thousands who are graduates of programs that specialize in nutrition. A change of eating pattern provides longer sustained energy and relief from headaches, tension, and emotional extremes. It stops the roller coaster effect of a high blood sugar level followed by an extreme drop, which often produces a craving sensation. This nonspecific craving, often experienced after consumption of foods high in sugar content, can lead to relapse and a return to chemical use. Many nutritionists working with recovering alcoholics have found that the frequent meals, packed with nutritious food substances, will allow the body to mend and the mind and emotions to stabilize. This new way of eating, combined with exercise and relaxation and following a thorough detoxification process, provides for good, solid physical recovery. When this dimension is well established, the other four dimensions are much easier to develop and sobriety easier to maintain. Physical recovery must be a priority in sobriety. It can provide the relief that many have been in search of for years.

DIMENSION NO. 2: MENTAL

Mental recovery is a gradual process of renewing the mind after years of negative and destructive thoughts. It refers strictly to the thinking process of the brain; feelings and emotions are covered in the section on emotional recovery that follows. When mental recovery occurs, the person regains judgment, makes positive decisions, and is able to communicate effectively. This aspect of recovery is based on an individual's ability to reprogram the mind and completely alter a faulty or negative thinking process. Built upon the foundation of a strong physical recovery, it becomes a key to emotional healing and resolution of problems with feelings. Before the feelings can be corrected, the thoughts must be reversed.

Replacing Negative Thoughts

To change a destructive mind and thoughts, new information must be fed into the mind. This information must cover new ways of considering the addiction problem and of viewing life. The addict is not privy to accurate information while still using or drinking. The information received is severely distorted. The first distortion is that of the delusions produced by the chemical.

The chemicals alter the mood and the mind so that what is perceived as reality is something much different. The other distortion is that of denial. The only information the addict will cling to is what supports denial of the problem. If the addict reads some drug article which states that addicts look like penguins, then he or she will clip and keep that article as sure proof that addiction has been avoided.

Denial perverts the information that is provided to the addict or alcoholic, who often distorts it to avoid facing the need to change. For example, some would take the material on heredity in Chapter Four and use it as an excuse to not change. They might think or even say, "See, I was born this way, so there is nothing I can do about it." The correct way to use that information would be to say, "Since I was born this way, others have been born this way. It was not my fault. I did not cause it. But others have changed, so I can change. I must accept the responsibility to change. No one will do it for me." In mental recovery, all information is used to point toward the tremendous hope for change rather than the despair found in feelings of helplessness.

There are many ways to acquire information that will reprogram the mind. One of the best is going to hear a recovering alcoholic or addict share what happened, how recovery became reality. This reinforces the fact that the alcoholic or addict is not alone, that others have made it through to the hope of recovery. These talks can also provide insight into how to put together a solid recovery plan. There is hope found in the messages of recovery of others. Alcoholics Anonymous holds regular speakers' meetings, which afford many opportunities to hear miraculous stories of recovery. The talks provide valuable information that helps the alcoholic think in a new way, being reminded both of the progression of addiction, and of the hope for change. This inspiration and motivation, combined with the new information, make attendance at speakers' meetings a dynamic plus in recovery.

There are other sources of information in addition to speakers' meetings: lectures, books, and tapes on addiction, alcoholism, and recovery. All are helpful in the rethinking process and provide a basis for the recovering person to refocus mentally. To salvage a lifetime of negative and destructive thinking, the mind must constantly be bombarded, even saturated, with new information. As new facts begin to take root in a person's mind, new attitudes emerge. These attitudes are what carry the person into the daily recovery process and the relief that it provides. When patients of a hospital-based program are awakened each morning, they begin a program designed to completely change their thinking. They are approached from every available angle to assist in developing attitudes helpful in sobriety. One source of information builds on another. Lectures are followed by discussion groups that reinforce the material presented. Reading assignments are made more understandable with the help of cassette and videotapes. Every component is designed to change the thinking and assist the addict in forming new and helpful attitudes. Without new information to replace the old, recovery is a more needlessly difficult task.

New information must be accompanied by the abandonment of unhealthy old thoughts and ideas. The subtle sources of negative information should be avoided. Movies and television series are full of role models and situations that reinforce the acceptance of addiction and drug use. Their subtle message is that "everyone is doing it." But everyone is not. These false depictions of life and alcohol and drug use can be depressing and reinforce the old attitudes that prevented recovery. Recovery is too precious to be destroyed by the negative influence of the media.

One way of countering the negative and reinforcing the positive is through the use of a journal. A journal can be a place to record helpful and positive insights into recovery; when memorable comments are heard or concepts discovered and written down, the journal can become a personal resource of courage and inspiration. It is so easy to forget helpful facts or ideas and principles; but when recorded in a journal, they are preserved for those times when they are most needed. They constitute a recovery manual designed to meet the individual's specific needs. A journal is a valuable recovery tool that costs nothing to maintain.

Replacing Negative "Friends"

Friends and acquaintances must not be ignored when considering the development of healthy thoughts and attitudes. Some people simply will fight everything new, good, or positive. They are so filled with their own hurts and problems that they cannot tolerate anyone else getting relief from theirs. They reinforce the negative and discard the positive. They question, badger, argue, and refute until the recovering person finally succumbs to their negative influence. They must be avoided. They have no place in a recovering person's life during the initial days of sobriety. Their influence can reverse the progress made through acceptance of new information.

To conclude, after the body is on a course toward recovery, the mind must be focused in the same direction. New information must be absorbed so that thoughts and attitudes become friends and allies in the recovery process. Whatever reinforces old negative thoughts and attitudes must be avoided and discarded. No book, movie, tape, television program, or friend is more valuable than recovery. Whatever stands in the way of developing a new mind must be replaced with support. Every aspect of the person's life must be in line with a new way of thinking that will allow an easier and more meaningful mental recovery.

DIMENSION NO. 3: EMOTIONAL

Emotional recovery is not possible unless physiological and mental recovery are under way. A central nervous system affected by extreme swings in blood sugar levels and constantly stimulated by caffeine and nicotine is not going to stabilize as well as when good nutritional principles are used, and someone who constantly steeps himself or herself in negative talk and negative information cannot hope to recover good, healthy emotions. The focus of the mind and the emotions must be unified. Confusion in one produces confusion in the other. To manage the emotions, body and mind must work together as a powerful recovery force.

No doubt the most painful area of recovery is the emotions. It is not fun to process negative feelings that have been suppressed or hidden for years. Often work in this area is avoided or delayed because of the pain associated with it, but it must be a part of recovery. In the midst of a forward-and-upward phase, time should be allowed for appropriate introspection. During this time the emotional skeletons in the closet are rattled, but once rattled and resolved, they can be put away, never to haunt again.

It's easier to remain a stoic who shares nothing of what is

happening inside than to open yourself for self-examination and reflection. Feelings do not have to be concealed; no macho manual makes it mandatory to hide and cover up emotional reality. People do not get well when they force back the uncomfortable feelings that must be addressed. It is known that cancer patients become much sicker when emotions such as anger and fear are suppressed. The barrier of unexpressed feelings hampers the process of living life to the fullest. The words of the song title "You Are Only as Sick as Your Secrets" are quite true. Hiding is not helpful; the hidden only grows in strength in its suppression. It surfaces, even stronger, at some later, more difficult time.

Assistance in Emotional Recovery

Emotional recovery can be accomplished only in relationships with other people; it cannot happen alone or in isolation. A group setting is mandatory. That group could be a recovery group, a self-help group, or a growth group. It could even, in some instances, be a supportive recovering family. Emotional growth is fostered by the power of a group. When the group is safe and supportive, the individual can explore feelings, express emotions, and resolve internal conflict. It becomes a source of support and fosters the acceptance of individual uniqueness. In a group, a recovering person has many consultants in the growth process. These people can reflect the reality needed to "ground" distorted emotions. In groups it is vital that people share and open up—and listen. In this environment, the addict or alcoholic is able to express thoughts and emotions authentically without the risk of rejection. Any time phoniness creeps in, the group can pierce the facade and usher the individual back to reality.

Failure in recovery is found in those who strive to *prove* their strength rather than *develop* strength. They want to be the exception and prove that recovery can be accomplished alone. In their times of greatest motivation and desire to change, they want to believe that it is only the will to change that is needed. Recovery cannot be accomplished alone; emotional growth will only be stifled in isolation. Even when alcoholics or addicts stop drinking and drugging, without the help of others they do not start growing. They remain emotionally immature and unbalanced. They must forsake the lonely struggle and reestablish relationships.

When a chemical provides instant gratification and instant relief from emotional pain, there is no chance for the user to mature. In chemical abuse, emotional growth and maturing are halted. That is why you hear forty-year-old addicts describe themselves as being fourteen emotionally. In a group, a person is encouraged to reverse the deterioration of maturity. Emotional development begins when the individual no longer runs from the pain but meets it head on, resolves it, and grows stronger from it. Talk to someone who is attempting recovery in isolation and you will understand the futility of recovery without relationships. Talk to someone who has reconnected, is a part of a group and a part of the real world, and you will find healthy growth and maturity.

One of the strongest components of the group dynamic is accountability. The healthiest and most helpful groups do not just sit around and discuss the past week. They focus on the need for a person to accept responsibility and take action. Rather than listen to the addict or alcoholic talk of the lack of support by a spouse, the group will focus on the person's need to foster that support. They might make an assignment for the individual to ask the spouse what could be done to achieve greater support. Or they might assign the person to make a date with the spouse. Then the group will follow up and make sure the assignment has been carried out. This accountability factor is missing from the recovery of too many people. It is good training for the time when the individual becomes self-accountable. Nothing fosters maturity better than accountability. Many people would rather walk on hot coals than be accountable to anyone, but once accountability is accepted, it allows authenticity and responsibility to flourish in a relationship.

One common thing that happens to almost every alcoholic or addict is the destruction of relationships. Along with this goes the destruction of accountability, allowing the problem to progress unchecked. For instance, witness the powerful executive surrounded by those who say only what he or she expects to hear. Isolated and unaccountable due to their position, such people have great difficulty in seeing the reality of the problem, and no one is willing to take the risk of confronting them with it. These people, as well as other addicts, must learn to accept accountability in recovery. Group accountability, especially in these difficult cases, is not enough but must be accompanied by individual accountability. Alcoholics Anonymous encourages the acceptance of a sponsor. The sponsor, who has "been there," has the right to tell the person to "shut up and listen." The sponsor can help the recovering person to learn to function in an accountable relationship. Then this ability can be transferred to other relationships with friends and family.

The most powerful aspect of accountability is the right to confront. Confrontation of denial that resurfaces in early recovery must occur instantly. When things begin to fall in place or start to look better, there is a great temptation for alcoholics or addicts to deny the extent of the problem. They want to believe that "I was not that bad yet" or "I'm certainly not as bad as some other people." The sponsor or the group can confront the person with the reality of the problem and the need for everything available in recovery. When denial starts to emerge, honesty in recovery is lost. For sobriety to be maintained, there must be complete honesty. Confrontation in an accountable relationship keeps the person honest; it restores the need to face reality, all of reality.

Beneath every person who is abusive and destructive while drinking and drugging lies a healthy individual waiting to emerge. Emotional recovery allows the unearthing of the real, positive person buried beneath the obsessions and compulsions. In emotional recovery, all compensation and fakery are abandoned. Emotional recovery is a return to the rare state of authenticity. The authentic person can accept self with all its weaknesses and strengths. He or she is able to identify real feelings and express those feelings appropriately. That unique individual is ready to be shared with others, and the dimension of social recovery can be developed.

DIMENSION NO. 4: SOCIAL

Recovery also demands some degree of ease with others. One cannot be comfortable with others when there is discomfort with oneself, so the person who is unhealthy emotionally will not be able fully to recover socially. Emotional strength is needed to face the world. Discomfort, inferiority, and self-imposed isolation mark a person struggling to recover socially on a foundation of emotional immaturity and insecurity. When social recovery is difficult, it is not a sign of failure; it simply means that the individual must return to a focus on emotional recovery. When the maturity process is developed, then social recovery becomes less of an everyday struggle.

Social recovery involves many different elements. It is more than just getting together with other people. It involves the ability to create an environment supportive of sobriety. The person who recovers socially sifts through the tangles of life to develop sincere, authentic relationships that will add to the quality of life rather than detract from it. Social recovery also involves developing activities that are positive, supportive, and conducive to sobriety. The individual attracted to a crowd must stop and ask some very important questions: "Who is in the crowd?" "Where is that crowd going?" "What will the crowd accomplish?" "Can I stay sober in the crowd?" Latching onto a crowd is not the same thing as developing a meaningful relationship. Just skipping from one group to the next, not relating, is far from social recovery. Social recovery involves the whole person—mind, body, and emotions—interacting comfortably with the people and places of a supportive environment.

Social Inventory

A helpful exercise is to take a social inventory. It can point out people, places, and things in the environment that are not conducive to recovery. It can also point to what is healthy in the social realm and what can be done to build on the strength of those healthy aspects. The answers for these twenty questions will constitute a useful social inventory:

1. With whom do I spend most of my time?
2. What do we do most often when we are together?
3. When we leave each other, has the time been healthy, or do I leave feeling a bit empty or guilty?
4. What do I do with my family?
5. How much of my time is spent in leisure activities with the family?
6. Am I involved with any groups outside the family?
7. Is my association with those groups constructive to my sobriety?
8. Who is consistently the most helpful and supportive person in my life?
9. Is my time with that person too limited?

10. Who in my life always seems to bring out the worst in me?
11. How often do I find myself trapped into spending time with that person?
12. Who are the people I have wanted to know better but haven't made the effort to know?
13. What are some supportive groups that I could join?
14. Where is the *un*healthiest place I go?
15. What can I do to substitute for time spent there?
16. Who appears interested in sharing a part of what I do, think, and feel?
17. What could I do to make opportunities for those caring people to share my world?
18. What defensive tactic do I use that prevents people from getting to know the real me?
19. In what circumstances and situations do I find it hardest to be myself?
20. Where do I feel most comfortable with myself and those around me?

When these questions are considered carefully, they can help in formulating a plan for complete social recovery. Being honest with oneself is essential for recovery. Being truthful about the inventory can identify areas that need the most change and improvement. There is one very important consideration to be made from the inventory, involving those people who are unsupportive and detrimental to the recovery process. Those people must be eliminated from day-to-day contact because of the negative social pressure they exert.

Changing Playmates and Playgrounds

Long ago, Alcoholics Anonymous identified the essence of social recovery, summing it up as the need to "change playmates and playgrounds." This entails avoiding those people who cannot adjust to the recovery of the alcoholic or addict. When a chemically dependent person starts to get well, it can be a threat to another's security. Such insecurity in someone else can unconsciously drive the addict or alcoholic toward relapse. This is especially true when old drinking buddies are faced with the recovery of one of their members. It forces them to look at their own drinking behavior and the results it has produced in their lives. They can attempt to chisel away at the stability of their exbuddy's recovery. This can be done with belittling questions like "How did you get on this recovery kick?" or "How long do you think this thing is going to last this time?" or, even more detrimental, "Now that the stress is gone, I'll bet you could handle a drink better than ever." And then there is the proverbial "Just one couldn't hurt." All these questions and comments are rooted in the insecurity of destructive people.

The process of eliminating the negative social pressure must be balanced. It is not an excuse for divorce, nor should friends and family, no matter how unhealthy they may be, be left out of the alcoholic's life forever. It often happens that a spouse who has grown sicker daily from the alcoholic's drinking is left or divorced after three months of sobriety, in the name of growth and recovery. Everyone needs time to get themselves together; that is why there can be such great value in staying in a halfway house during the initial days of sobriety. This allows everyone to grow and adjust in a less stressful atmosphere. It also provides incentive for the person who must grow, mature, and recover before returning home. Time away in the recovery home allows total support and accountability, which can be a welcome replacement for unhealthy friends. When recovery and sobriety are stable, old relationships can be mended and developed, but until then, it is best to replace unhealthy associations with destructive "playmates" with those that are 100 percent supportive of recovery and a new life.

As for "playgrounds," a bar is not the healthiest, most supportive place for an alcoholic, and a party where everyone is using drugs is not the place for a drug addict to hang out. Many playgrounds of the alcoholic and addict need changing. Any situation, hangout or establishment not conducive to healthy social recovery needs to be replaced. To continue to be in compromising situations is to flirt with disaster. There are certain areas that must be declared off-limits, out-of-bounds, and dangerous. This aspect of social recovery may be the key to long-term sobriety. A lifetime good-bye to unhealthy situations may be the best insurance for sobriety. Social recovery must involve protection from unhealthy people in unhealthy places.

To prevent a return to a life-style of isolation, the unhealthy environments should be replaced with healthy, supportive ones. If not, the addict or alcoholic will be confined to a life of a recluse. Cultivation of people and places that provide positive reinforcement must be a priority. The biggest problem is finding those supportive locations where recovery is reinforced. Churches, night classes, exercise clubs, health clubs, recovery groups, and Alcoholics Anonymous meetings are among the many settings that can replace negative situations.

Sharing life with others rather than hiding from those who want to grow close is the essence of social recovery. The value of relationships replaces the futility of a totally self-centered existence. There is an attitude change that moves a person out of the role of a taker and into that of a giver. A person who recovers socially looks for ways to contribute to society rather than to continually grab or rip it off. Social recovery also involves the healing and mending of old relationships and the development of new ones. When handled in the proper span of time, it becomes a process whereby a supportive network of people and places form an environment enabling recovery.

Social recovery is awkward. It requires practice and persistence. A group therapy or a recovery group setting can help in the resocialization process. The group can be a supportive environment where new behavior can be practiced and rehearsed. Interaction difficulties can be worked out before they affect relationships. The rough edges of self-determined living can be polished off in the group. This is the most helpful component of social recovery. Negative attitudes and behavior can be worked out in the group, enabling stronger relationships to be developed outside the group.

Human beings are social creatures. They need social recovery as much as any other type of recovery. For recovery to be complete, relationships, especially the close ones, must be healed. Sharing thoughts and feelings is a major portion of life. To be unable to do that is to miss a major portion of life. In the end, the person who does not recover socially does not recover at all.

DIMENSION NO. 5: SPIRITUAL

There is no area of recovery more controversial or more difficult to discuss in this book than the spiritual. No matter which approach is used, people will disagree about its appropriateness. The atheist or agnostic is most likely to view this section as too religious and reject its importance. Those who have grown and

matured spiritually may find the material weak and noncom-
mittal. The Christian is likely to ask, "Where is Jesus in all
this?" Remember that people are at very different places in their
spiritual journey. Those much farther along in the journey must
understand how difficult this area is for those who have for years
felt alienated from God and often been on the outs with religious
institutions or anything connected with church. A large degree
of acceptance rather than judgment is necessary when helping
the alcoholic or addict with spiritual growth. The important concept of spiritual growth is that no matter where you are on the
spiritual journey, spiritual recovery will bring you closer to, and
ultimately involved with, the truth.

Some shy away from the spiritual growth dimension because
they want no part of anything remotely associated with religion.
Spiritual growth has nothing to do with religion. It involves the
facilitation of spiritual maturation. The fact that some religion
has lost the mission of helping people grow spiritually, or some
organization has stood in the way of growth, does not mean that
a person can afford to avoid spiritual growth. If one will look
hard enough, there is within almost every religious organization
or church people who are genuinely spiritually mature and can
assist in spiritual recovery. When a religion or church can assist
in the spiritual growth process, it is a great benefit for the alcoholic or addict to belong.

In many recovery groups you will find a lack of emphasis on
the importance of church in the recovery process. This is because of past rejection of people who had alcohol or drug problems. Those attitudes are changing within most churches. Those
who once alienated and rejected now welcome the alcoholic and
addict and often provide special recovery groups for them. When
a recovering person finds the right church with the right people
in it, it can be a tremendous source of support. Remember, the
problem has never been with religion or the church but with
those individuals who have distorted the church's mission and
used the church for selfish motives and the furtherance of am-
bition. Such problems with religion and church are often the
reason people are afraid or unwilling to recover spiritually. Many
alcoholics and addicts associate the church and religion with
spirituality. The attitudes about one are deeply rooted in the
attitudes about the other. The addict or alcoholic must move

beyond this barrier, not use past attitudes as an excuse to remain spiritually stagnant.

Frequently people will "get religious" and believe they are growing spiritually. They merely improve their respectability by wrapping the church and religion around themselves. What may result, rather than spiritual growth, is a form of compensation that produces religiosity or religious fanaticism. Looking better or attempting to look better has nothing to do with spiritual growth. A spiritually mature individual possesses a congruency on the inside and outside. Anything that appears wonderful to the world must be sacrificed for whatever results in genuine internal spiritual growth.

The first step toward spiritual growth is the acknowledgment of a higher power. The alcoholic or addict must be willing to accept assistance from a being with greater power than the individual. The term *higher power* is offensive to some who believe it is a diluted way of addressing God. Of course, the Christian questions why Christ is not acknowledged. He or she must accept that acknowledgment of a higher power is only a beginning. It is at the start of a search for truth. In addition, higher power is a term that is important for recovery. There are a lot of people who may believe in God, or even Christians who believe in Christ, who do not allow God or Christ to be a power greater or higher than themselves. They acknowledge God's existence with lip service and continue to run their lives without the assistance of a higher power. Tapping into your own power reserves is not the result or purpose of spiritual growth.

When God really is acknowledged and accepted as God, then God will be allowed to act and interact in the person's life with power to do those things beyond the grasp of individual effort. Many frustrations will no longer be fought, but instead turned over to God. No ego, will, or conceit must be allowed to stand in the way of what a person and God can do together. Those accomplishments may not be seen by the world on the outside, but they will be experienced by the person on the inside.

The term higher power is also significant for anyone who is a proclaimed atheist. If in the beginning that person refuses to acknowledge God as real, for recovery to begin there must at least be the acknowledgment of something more powerful than the individual. The atheist may be able to accept only that the support group is a higher power, but at least the journey can start there. Rarely will a person stick to the group as the only power greater than himself or herself. In almost every case the person will eventually accept the reality of God as "the" higher power.

A book called *Recovery Without God*, full of stories of those who have attempted it, would be a very sad volume. When a person attempts recovery alone, failure results. Recurring relapse is frequently due to the weakness of the spiritual growth process because of an unwillingness to acknowledge God. If spiritual growth does not occur, other recovery dimensions will deteriorate. Those who remain skeptical about God usually remain miserable.

Spiritual recovery is a process of completion. Through spiritual recovery, the value of the individual, personal relationships, and the family can be restored. Guilt, fear, and anger vanish. Hope replaces despair; priorities change; life, lived with God's wisdom and not from a limited view of momentary self-gratification, has purpose and meaning. The natural, genuine person emerges—the person once covered by defensive barriers and denial. In spiritual recovery, the person finds the freedom to be real.

When the spiritual is combined with the other dimensions, the recovering alcoholic or addict is able to experience all the opportunities of life that everyone deserves and enjoys. Recovery must involve discipline, which is often painful. The discipline of recovering in all five areas is like the tension on a string that enables the kite to soar above the earth. It is the discipline within the recovery system that allows freedom and hope to grow rather than diminish. All five areas must be developed in disciplined perspective to each other. One dimension can never be ignored to allow some other dimension to become the complete focus of recovery.

No matter how long a person has been drinking or taking drugs, recovery in all five dimensions is the answer. No one should delay implementing changes in all five areas by looking for the source of the problem or the "reasons why." Recovery is available to anyone willing to change and become a complete, whole person. Recovery cannot happen alone. There are plenty of resources to assist in the recovery process; treatment centers, outpatient programs, counselors, and self-help programs have worked for years to help people start over, as discussed in the previous chapter. Once the willingness to recover is there, help is available. The beginning of a completely new life can start by the simple act of reaching out to someone for help. That effort can be made today.

CHAPTER TWELVE

RELAPSE

Dana Miller had been a heavy drinker and drug user during her college years. She was an addict in every way. She wanted and needed some mood-altering chemical every day. Twice her mother had to pick her up at the U.C.L.A. Medical Center because of a bad trip from LSD. She had tried virtually everything. Most people would not have given her any chance for recovery. But, amazingly, she did recover.

Recovery began when Dana "hit bottom." And just as she had abused drugs in a big way, she hit bottom in a big way also. It happened during her senior year in college. She and three of her friends were driving over to some condominiums in Newport Beach after an evening of booze and cocaine. When the cocaine was gone, they continued their binge with pot. They were going to settle in at the place of a guy who went to school with them, but they never made it there.

Dana was driving north on Pacific Coast Highway in Newport Beach, headed for Superior Avenue. Her male friend lived just at the top of Superior, which winds upward about three hundred feet from the Pacific Coast Highway. Dana turned onto Superior and made her way toward the top of the hill. On her right was a drop-off unprotected by a fence or shrubs of any kind. As she reached the top, a car coming from the opposite direction swerved into her lane. She jerked the wheel to the right, sending her car down the three-hundred-foot drop. When it hit the bottom, all of the girls were screaming and scratching to find a way out of the car—all of them except Dana's best friend, in the front passenger seat. She was dead.

The following months were full of depositions, court appearances, and a very important event for Dana's defense. She went into treatment for alcohol and drug addiction. The death of her friend and the legal process of facing charges of involuntary manslaughter brought Dana to the end of her alcohol and drug use and to the beginning of the recovery process. She did well in treatment and established a strong recovery program. She set out to live her life free of alcohol and drugs, one day at a time.

Dana served no time for the death of her friend. Her lawyer had managed to get her a three-year probation, with several hundred hours of community service, in exchange for a plea of guilty. If she drank or used drugs, she would be brought back before the judge and sentenced to prison. But Dana was not chiefly motivated by the desire to stay out of prison. She really wanted to start her life anew. She set out to build an enduring sobriety. She wanted a life full of meaning and purpose.

Dana finished school two years after the accident. She obtained a degree in social work and went to work at the Free Clinic in Laguna Beach. She married a man she met at a church-sponsored singles' retreat. They settled in a small house in Laguna. It appeared that everything was going their way, that Dana had captured the life that had passed her by for so many years. She had no desire to drink or drug again. All she wanted was to continue her work at the clinic and start a family soon. For once in her life, she could honestly say that she was happy.

It did not happen suddenly but was instead a gradual easing away from recovery and into relapse. Dana started skipping her Wednesday night and Friday morning AA meetings. She convinced her husband that all that was behind her. She knew in her heart that she would never do drugs again. She also stopped seeing the friends who had helped her in the early days of her recovery. All the people and activities that had been helpful in her recovery began to drop out of her life.

This did not alarm her husband. He felt that she had probably matured beyond the point of needing a recovery support system. In fact, he was pleased to have more of her time. He welcomed the evenings at home with her; he felt they had been too cluttered with recovery meetings, recovery lectures, and recovering friends.

There were other things that dropped out of Dana's life. She quit going to work out at the health club; she was not motivated to exercise. And she no longer watched her eating habits. Dana filled her stomach with sweets; all the ice cream she had resisted was eaten in a couple of months. Her weight soared out of control.

After a period without the recovery support system she had been used to, Dana's attitude deteriorated further. She began to wonder if she might be able to drink socially. She was convinced that drugs had done her in, but she was not so sure about alcohol. She knew that she had been fully addicted, but that was several years back. She felt that now, older, wiser, and more mature, she would not find drinking a problem. At least not one or two drinks.

She began to call up some of her old drinking and drugging friends. She would meet them in Huntington Beach, and they would go to some of the places familiar from their college days. Dana did not drink or use, but she said she was lonely for her old friends; she wanted to laugh with them again and relive some of the old times. She wanted to talk about the fun times and go to the fun places. She was still not drinking or using, but the question of whether she could or not occupied her thoughts more urgently each day.

Finally, after a week of difficult cases at work and some strained arguments with her husband, she took her first drink in six years. She met a friend at a local bar, and they both drank until two o'clock in the morning. Her friend took her home to her husband, who immediately knew that she had been drinking. The next day was full of promises that it would never happen again. She told him she had answered the question of whether or not she could drink socially; she knew and accepted that she could not. She said that she would now be able to be abstinent forever. But she was wrong.

Fortunately for Dana, her husband was not willing for her drinking to continue. He knew that she had progressed through the complete gamut of relapse. So he drove her back to the treatment center where she had first received help for her drinking and drugs. It was there that her long-term sobriety began. Her husband, fully active in the treatment process, was determined to help her out of the relapse and back into the recovery that had allowed them to meet and marry. Together they developed a recovery plan to help her stay off drugs and alcohol and to stay involved with all the people and activities that supported her recovery. Three years and two children later, she was well on her way to obtaining the life that she deserved. As far as I know, her recovery remains strong.

The relapse process that happened to Dana happens to thousands of recovering alcoholics and drug addicts every year. Alcoholism, like heart disease, is a relapsing disease. Relapse can happen after many years of sobriety or it can begin the first day the addict goes without alcohol or drugs. Relapse is not merely the return to an addictive chemical but a process that happens in progressive stages. Relapse is a direct opposite to the process of recovery and ultimately ends in the decompensation of the addict and loss of control. The decompensation results in the use of the addictive chemical, nervous breakdown, repeated accidents, and physical or emotional collapse. In relapse, the symptoms of illness reemerge and take complete control of the person's life.

For the alcoholic, alcohol has been a source of self-treatment for years. That self-treatment becomes a life-style, an unsuccessful way of life. Recovery must replace self-treatment with the acceptance of help from others. There must be a continual process of looking beyond self to God and others for assistance. When the focus returns to a self-treatment mentality and a self-assured abstinence, the relapse process begins.

The intensity of relapse varies from person to person. Some return to uncontrolled drinking quickly and continue to drink for years. Others reverse relapse before drinking or drugging ever starts. The difference is usually made by the significant others around the person in relapse. If they act decisively and quickly, the relapse can be reversed before damage is extreme. They are the key to helping the addict in relapse return to the point where recovery starts. That point is the reestablishment of a willingness to do whatever it takes, a willingness to do everything possible to establish and maintain sobriety.

Initially, recovery for the alcoholic begins when he or she understands and accepts that alcohol is the problem. Since alcohol is the problem, the only way to continue recovery is to remain totally abstinent, and to keep abstinence as a priority, the alcoholic knows that a recovery program is necessary. It is the only way to maintain abstinence, improve quality of life, and build supportive relationships. The recovering alcoholic is willing to do whatever it takes to keep these priorities as the focal point of living. Relapse begins when they fade as priorities. Relapse ends when significant others and family members help the alcoholic reestablish them. Just as it is unproductive to wait for the alcoholic to start recovery alone, it is unproductive to expect the alcoholic to reverse the relapse process alone.

Those in the field of alcoholism treatment see the evidence of relapse every day. Alcohol and drug treatment centers see patients readmitted after a drinking binge or drugging spree, and alongside those patients come the family members whose hopes have been dashed on empty bottles or syringes. Alcoholics Anonymous regularly welcomes members back into the fold who have "slipped," the term they use for relapse. AA celebrates more birthdays or anniversaries of a year of sobriety in January than at any other time. Probably this reflects the large number of people who relapse over the Christmas and New Year's holidays. The holiday blues and stresses of family relationships take their toll on sobriety. Relapse is part of the recovery process for most, and frequently results in a return to drinking, or taking drugs.

Relapse does not always mean resuming the addiction. It can be manifested in bizarre accidents or being accident-prone. For some the relapse process results in a state of total misery, in which life becomes less manageable than when the drinking was an everyday part of it. Divorce will often signal that a relapse has happened, even though drinking has not resumed. A marriage that survived twenty years of drinking finds difficulty surviving six months without alcohol when the alcoholic is not recovering but is in some stage of relapse.

One man returned to treatment after almost a year without any drugs or alcohol. An extremely rigid man, he returned only at the threat of a brother who said he would have him committed to a mental institution otherwise. Counselling him and his wife revealed an almost unbelievable picture of that year without alcohol. When he arrived home from treatment, his bizarre behavior began immediately. He took a felt pen and wrote the date of his last drink on the living room wall. Every day he went without alcohol, he placed a mark by that date, marking the days as if he were a prisoner, captive in a lonely cell. He would frequently drag his wife or children to that spot to stare at the date with him. The month before he returned to the hospital, his behavior escalated to a stage of potential homicide. He would come home from work, go to the tool shed and grab his ax, then sit in front of the television set, expecting to be waited on for the entire evening. The sad thing was that his wife was willing to exist this way for so long. She took action only after he threatened to chop off his children's heads when they did not bring home all A's. This man never drank, but he was in complete relapse. He never began the recovery process. He was in relapse from the first day he quit drinking.

This type of relapse occurs frequently and is rarely identified as such. Most people think relapse is a return to the chemical of choice, but relapse begins long before the chemical use returns, and frequently chemical use is not part of it. There are many symptoms that point to a "dry drunk" or chemical-free relapse. Stress-related illness is often a red flag that signals the relapse process. Heart disease, colitis, migraines, ulcers, and nervous disorders in the supposedly recovering alcoholic are signs of relapse; so are catastrophes such as accidents, divorce, or suicide attempts. Frequently severe depression will totally incapacitate the individual. A collapse, either physical or emotional, signals that the alcoholic, whether drinking or not, is in relapse and in need of help.

One of the reasons for relapse being a part of so many recoveries is the central nervous system. The central nervous system does not heal immediately. It is not uncommon to see the effects of a sick central nervous system two or three years after the drinking or drugs stop. The delicate nerve fibers have been damaged from years of chemical abuse, either saturated with the addictive chemicals or suffering withdrawal from them. Healing from such abuse takes time, and until it is complete, the alcoholic experiences varying degrees of emotional and mental augmentation. Essentially, because of the sensitivity of that delicate but sick nervous system, the emotions are intensified for the alcoholic. It is as if an emotional volume control were turned up. The recovering person is in a constant battle trying to control emotional peaks and valleys that reach higher and fall deeper than for the normal person.

The sick central nervous system affects every area of mental and emotional functioning. Thinking is distorted, and problem solving is impaired. Memory is clogged, and the ability to react mentally is slowed. At the same time there is a tendency to overreact emotionally to the smallest of irritations. The emotional extremes are complicated by a sense of numbness that may overwhelm the person for days. All these symptoms, which leave the person attempting to recover overly stressed and fatigued, can be summed up as a *postwithdrawal* or *protracted withdrawal* syndrome. When it occurs, the recovery program must be stepped up and intensified. The recovering person must draw closer to the support system and ask for assistance from a sponsor, counselor, or friend. The individual may even need to return to the controlled environment of an inpatient treatment setting. If action is not taken in the time of acute postwithdrawal, a return to the chemical stimulation or sedation is almost guaranteed. Not understanding what is happening and not acting appropriately to counter it causes many people to relapse.

Another factor probably contributes to more relapses than a slowly healing central nervous system or one that is in protracted withdrawal. The chief reason that people relapse is the difference between reality and the expectations of the recovering alcoholic. If the individual expects an easy recovery, achieved without effort, relapse will occur. Recovery is difficult, and the recovering alcoholic must accept that as reality and act accordingly. He or she must not expect early rewards for stopping drinking. The rewards will come after a solid life-style of positive rewards is established, and after the entire body has had a chance to heal completely. Rather than looking for early rewards, the newly recovering alcoholic must establish a system of protection from the internal and external demands of early recovery.

Reality, at times, is not very exciting. Reality sometimes includes a family that was expecting an instant cure. This type of family places extra demands on the alcoholic trying to recover from years of alcohol and drug abuse. A recovering person must not count on total support from a healthy family. The more likely reality is a lowered ability to handle the stress of an overly demanding family. Because of the long healing process, the early days of recovery are often more difficult than the days of drinking. If the alcoholic's expectation is one of reduced stress and less difficulty, relapse will set in early. For recovery to be long-term, expectations, especially early expectations, must be based on reality. When reality is ignored, relapse results.

Relapse destroys families. The longer it lasts, the more destructive it becomes. Identification of its early symptoms is vital for early intervention. When intervention is successful, the alcoholic, drifting hopelessly through relapse, is given the opportunity to start over. Often the hope for the recovering alcoholic rests in the hands of family members who can identify symptoms of relapse and take action. The other hope is for the recovering alcoholic to know what to expect in early recovery, and to know the early warning signs of relapse.

Relapse occurs in a predictable progression which has four phases or stages. The intensity and duration of each phase vary for everyone. Each time a person drinks again, the other stages have been completed. The progression begins with the first stage, *complacency*. Complacency forms the foundation of the entire destructive progression. Whether or not the end result is a return to drinking, relapse is in full progress when complacency sets in.

FIRST STAGE OF RELAPSE: COMPLACENCY

Complacency is easily identified. It starts when the recovering person stops doing those things that were designed to improve the quality of life, particularly going to Alcoholics Anonymous, Narcotics Anonymous, or some other recovery group. Aftercare meetings are abandoned; counselor or therapist appointments are no longer kept. These activities stop because denial grows, killing the motivation for recovery.

Some statements are clear demonstrations of denial:

"I don't need to go to AA anymore."

"I know I will never drink again."

"I don't need counseling."

"I'm doing better than ever."

"I don't need anyone to help me now."

"I don't need to work the steps."

"I'm so involved with helping others, I don't have time for all I used to do."

"I don't have a problem now."

The complacent alcoholic denies the problem and denies needs. That person will deny feelings and emotions rather than deal with them and process them, will ignore fear of failure instead of discussing it with a sponsor or counselor. When the alcoholic stops addressing problems and denies that they exist, complacency and relapse have replaced recovery.

The denial so obvious in complacency is usually accompanied by overconfidence. The overconfidence is totally unfounded; when it takes over, the recovering person is usually at the point of greatest vulnerability. There is a complete attitude change. When the attitude is correct, the recovering alcoholic will say, "I won't drink *today*." But the attitude of the overconfident addict in relapse is "I don't have to do anything today about my problems or recovery." The false belief that abstinence is all that is needed takes the place of a recovery program.

During complacency, the alcoholic stops planning for success. Living "one day at a time" should form the foundation of a future full of rewards and well-being, but the complacent alcoholic no longer lives a day at a time or plans appropriately. Planning is replaced by idleness and daydreaming. Wishful thinking is the only link to a future that will never be, establishing a world of fantasy that becomes a flight from reality. It is a futile existence of unfulfilled expectations and unrealistic dreams. The alcoholic appears to be dazed and immobile, fighting and trying not to lose ground while losing ground every day.

The alcoholic also becomes very defensive about his or her recovery. Just as alcohol was an avoided subject before recovery began, any part of the recovery program is now off-limits for conversation. The alcoholic rationalizes away any evidence that recovery is at a standstill. The defensiveness is extremely pronounced at this point of irresponsibility. The alcoholic wants people to believe that things are better than ever, that all is under control. When the reality is presented that an irresponsible lifestyle is being established, the alcoholic will maintain doggedly that he or she is unlike other alcoholics or drug addicts who have stopped using chemicals.

One last example of the complacency stage is self-analysis. The alcoholic will claim to have greater self-insight. When reliance on external support stops, the alcoholic begins self-analysis and brooding. This delving into self is a narcissistic attempt to justify withdrawal and isolation from others. The more the alcoholic looks inward, the less action is taken; it is just an excuse, an intellectualized reason, for discontinuing recovery. Self-analysis is a major sign that the alcoholic has returned to the "stinking thinking" of "I can handle it alone."

To sum up, in the complacency stage of relapse, whatever was healthy starts to erode from the recovery process. Poor eating habits replace regular eating patterns emphasizing protein and complex carbohydrates; nutrition is no longer a priority. Regular exercise is also abandoned, and the alcoholic refuses to make time for the most natural forms of stimulation and relaxation. Late nights and broken sleep replace regular times of rest. And of course, attendance at recovery meetings ends. All that was designed to improve the recovering alcoholic's quality of life is discontinued. The complacent alcoholic veers off the track leading to a life full of purpose and meaning and moves toward a life of frustration and misery.

SECOND STAGE OF RELAPSE: CONFUSION

The misery is intensified in the second stage of relapse, *confusion*. The alcoholic, disconnected from the support needed in recovery, begins to question the extent of the problem and whether the addiction was real. The "Am I or not?" thoughts and questions become obsessions that cloud other thoughts for hours. These are accompanied by questions of "Do I need to or not?" The alcoholic is confused about the need for abstinence, sobriety, counseling, AA, and support of all kinds. The question of the need for sobriety is coupled with the doubt about the ability to maintain sobriety. Confusion reigns in the alcoholic's mind and replaces the direction that guided recovery.

Problems for the confused alcoholic become bigger than life. Their proportions are exaggerated by the confusion. The alcoholic has difficulty in solving even the simplest of problems, at times seeing them as unsolvable. Extreme confusion blocks constructive, logical thinking. Self-esteem is lowered as self-doubt increases. The alcoholic feels incompetent at living, since the small problems are so hard to handle. As the alcoholic doubts himself or herself, the doubting carries over into other areas.

One of the most destructive doubts of the alcoholic in the confusion stage concerns the disease concept of alcoholism. The alcoholic doubts that it is a disease, and rationalizes that the alcohol-related problems were a part of a crisis or a temporary stage. There is tremendous doubt about whether the alcohol would produce the same results now that greater insight has been gained. Growth of the alcoholic's irrational feelings of omnipotence leads to the belief that the alcohol problem has been conquered, that anything is possible, and that no problem is beyond the alcoholic's scope.

The confusion stage is characterized by statements made to oneself and others:

"I don't think my problem was *that* bad."

"If it was a disease, I must be over it by now."

"If alcohol was the problem, then why am I so miserable without it?"

"I don't think anyone can help me with my problems; I'm different from the rest."

"Is *this* what people call happy?"

The confused alcoholic suffers from a growing depression. The depression increases as more and more expectations turn into false hopes. But the person has a hard time figuring out the source of the depression. Any existing plans begin to fail; nothing works out, and the depression and disappointment intensify. Total dissatisfaction characterizes the alcoholic's feeling about life. Since the "here and now" becomes so difficult to accept, the alcoholic chooses to live in the "there and then." The escape into unreality is an attempt to relieve the depression. The alcoholic longs for happiness but does not really know what it is and has a growing doubt that it will ever be felt again. In the midst of it all, the alcoholic will continue to try to persuade himself or herself and everyone else that all is well and everything is under control.

The alcoholic is anything but under control. The thinking process is totally distorted. Thoughts are filled with misperceptions about people, sobriety, and the stability of recovery. Irrational and inconsistent behavior results from distorted thinking and judgment. The words and actions of the alcoholic, confused and depressed, become unpredictable. In this stage some family members unconsciously help the alcoholic return to drinking. The reason is the predictability issue; when drinking, the alcoholic is more predictable than when in the confused stage. Not knowing what will happen next, not knowing how the person will react or behave from day to day, becomes more difficult to tolerate than drinking at its worst. So the emotions of the alcoholic's family are as out of control as the alcoholic's behavior. The state of confusion within the alcoholic is paralleled by the family's confusion. With so much confusion, doubt, and inconsistency, the next stages of relapse cannot be prevented unless someone takes action to reverse the progression.

THIRD STAGE OF RELAPSE: COMPROMISE

The third stage in the relapse progression is *compromise*. The complacent and confused alcoholic eventually starts to do things and go places that present extreme risks. These risky actions needlessly expose the person to the chemical that triggered the disease. Rather than continuing protective avoidance of drinking and drugging environments, the alcoholic or addict begins to ease back into these settings. The needless exposure to the pressure to use and drink again is the final compromising of the integrity of the recovery process.

When recovery was initiated, one of the key changes was in where the alcoholic went and with whom he or she spent time. The people and places for sobriety were positive and supportive of recovery, but that changes in this third phase of compromise. The old "playmates and playgrounds" are back. The alcoholic returns to those places and does those thing most dangerous to recovery. The life-style of the person seems to blur back into the same realm as when the heavy drinking was continuing. The only difference between the alcoholic now and then is that then there was drinking; now, the drinking has not started—yet.

For the relapsing alcoholic, life is defeat piled upon defeat. It was growing more unmanageable every day while drinking; now, without alcohol, it is also moving in an uncontrollable direction. The alcoholic's "black cloud" has returned. Nothing seems to work out as hoped; other people are not doing what is expected. The alcoholic wants people to cater, pamper, and meet needs, but the alcoholic's needs are so overwhelming that no one can meet them. Instead of people making life easier, each person is just another source of irritation, so the alcoholic breaks off many relationships and creates further barriers that separate him or her from support sources. As isolation grows, the alcoholic continues to fight and struggle, but with greater futility.

The alcoholic is not a happy person. He or she wishes for happiness but does not have a plan or support to find or achieve it. Everything seems to increase the alcoholic's anger and dissatisfaction. These feelings, piled on top of depression and periods of great anxiety, prompt the alcoholic to look for relief. There is a marked increase in the use of nonprescription drugs. That only lasts until the person turns to a physician to provide stronger relief than over-the-counter drugs can provide. The alcoholic becomes obsessed with the thoughts of social drinking. The question of whether the drinking can be controlled is repeated over and over in the alcoholic's mind. In the end, the need for relief is so intense that the alcoholic becomes convinced that just one drink would not hurt, but the drink is not consumed until every other alternative for relief has been tried.

In accepting the belief that a return to alcohol would not be a disaster, the alcoholic has committed the ultimate dishonest act and now continues to lie and deceive everyone. Recovery is an honesty program, and without honesty, it has no meaning at all. Once people close to the alcoholic sense that deception has returned, they tend to give up on him or her. If they confront the alcoholic about the lies and drastic deterioration in the quality of life, the confrontation is met with blaming, excuses, and projection. The alcoholic refuses to accept responsibility for the problems but instead tries to convince the confronters that they are the real problem, that if only *they* would change, everything would be better.

That "if only" statement is one of many "if onlys" the dishonest and irrational alcoholic uses. Others are:

"If only *you* could see the real problem."

"If only I had drunk just on the weekend."

"If only my parents had not been so rough on me."

"If only I had a beer, I'd feel better. And it would not be as bad as hard liquor."

All the "if only" statements demonstrate the ultimate compromise: honesty. Once the alcoholic compromises truth for fantasy and wishful thinking, the possibility of growth and maturity diminishes.

As the focus shifts from the alcoholic's own problems, some interesting methods are used to disguise the deterioration. The alcoholic steps up efforts to "work others' programs" and impose sobriety on anyone who drinks. The relapsing alcoholic becomes an expert on anything that relates to alcohol and drugs. And the "expertise" is shared obnoxiously with anyone who is willing to listen. All this is projection onto other people in an attempt to avoid and escape confronting the problems multiplying in the alcoholic's life.

The compromise stage is also full of impulsive behavior. No structure is left, and the alcoholic acts and reacts on a whim rather than according to a plan. The lack of daily structure results from an "I don't care" attitude. Since the alcoholic does not care about self or others or recovery, everything is okay to do. Rational decision-making is not called on to determine a course of action. Without thinking, the person resigns the job; relationships are broken impulsively; and other relationships are begun, most of them unhealthy. Living with this impulsive behavior is like living with a manic-depressive personality; when the consequences of the near-manic impulsive frenzy are felt, depression results, and the alcoholic continues to bounce from impulsive reaction to depression.

In a last-ditch effort to maintain sobriety or sanity, the alcoholic often radically compensates for his or her problems, sometimes with an unrealistic drive toward overworking. After a flare-up of compulsive workaholism, the compensation might prompt compulsive sports activities, like running or weight lifting. Other compulsive behaviors flourish: nonstop talking, lying, stealing, or gambling could all be part of this phase. The compulsive behaviors are unconscious efforts to cope, but they do not provide satisfaction or help the situation improve. They only lower the alcoholic's self-esteem even further. The helpless feeling becomes overwhelming as the alcoholic feels powerless, no matter what he or she has tried. Signs of self-pity are once again seen by family members and significant others. Resentments taint every relationship, whether with the family or at work. It seems that there is no end to the misery of the compromising alcoholic.

Toward the end of the compromise stage, the alcoholic experiences a great deal of apprehension about the future and his or her well-being. There is no pleasure in living, and anything that could possibly be fun is avoided. People who appear to be having fun are resented. Loneliness and isolation are the only company for the alcoholic. The fantasies about the enjoyment of social drinking absorb a lot of the alcoholic's idle time. It becomes evident that he or she is either going to drink again or that some other catastrophe will come along to rob the person of any control. Sometimes the alcoholic, sensing disaster, begins to hoard money and unconsciously prepare for the imminent collapse. This is the last major indicator of the compromise stage, warning that the fourth stage is not far off. Without intervention from family, friends, or employer, it is guaranteed to happen; no one remains mired in the compromise stage.

FOURTH STAGE OF RELAPSE: CATASTROPHE

The fourth and last stage of relapse is *catastrophe*. Catastrophe can occur in different forms. It can be a physical exhaustion that hospitalizes the person, emotional exhaustion, or a nervous breakdown. A psychiatric break or severe psychotic episode is another form of fourth-stage relapse. Anything that ultimately leaves the person incapacitated is a catastrophe. Suicide attempts, accidents, or illnesses all fall into this category, but the most common form of catastrophe is a return to the use of mood-altering drugs.

Often this final relapse stage is triggered. Looking back, it can be observed that one specific thing proved to be too much for the alcoholic and thrust the person into the catastrophe stage. The trigger could be an event: a positive event like the birth of a child or a negative event like being fired or being charged with drunk driving. An anniversary or birthday may trigger the catastrophe; holidays, especially Christmas and New Year's, are triggers for many alcoholics. During these times it is important for every alcoholic to be extra careful and protective, whether in relapse or recovery. Triggers can also come from less specific sources without exact dates. Times of high stress or reliving a bad memory can serve to trigger the alcoholic out of the compromise stage and into the catastrophe stage.

The return to chemical stimulation or sedation is usually the first point of recognizable relapse to those who are uneducated about the relapse process. It is first noted as controlled drinking or using. People may express amazement at the fact that the alcoholic can now control the drinking or the addict the drug use. The alcoholic may show signs of mood elevation as he or she proves that controlled drinking or using can be achieved after all. This is a short-lived victory; eventually all control is lost.

The loss of control usually does not happen immediately. It, like the relapse, happens in phases or stages. First, the alcoholic tries to maintain control by controlling the amount or quantity. The alcoholic will often set a definite limit and fight to maintain it, but the limit does not remain constant. The original limit might be three beers, and the person may go a couple of weeks drinking only three beers a day. But then he or she will want to drink more and try to stop at four beers. This continues until the limit is extended to five, then six—and then no limit can be maintained. But the person may not lose complete control and will try other methods.

When limiting the quantity fails, the alcoholic may resort to maintaining control by changing the type of alcohol consumed. The beer drinker resorts to light beer, the light beer drinker resorts to low-alcohol beer, the wine drinker may switch to beer or vice versa. And of course, the hard liquor drinker will choose wine or beer. The switch method will even involve changing brands; anything in the alcoholic's mind that will help him or her stay in control is used. But the efforts are futile. The end result is not sobriety.

When setting limits and changing types and brands fail, the alcoholic has no choice but self-imposed periods of abstinence. The alcoholic picks a time segment when no alcohol will be consumed and tries to stick to it. It could be a month or a week, but eventually the person has a hard time not drinking for one day. This stopping is not accompanied by any life-style enhancement at all; it is just another attempt to prove control even as control continues to dwindle.

Sooner or later the alcoholic must seek external help to live for any period without alcohol. He or she simply cannot make it without alcohol in the system. The person resorts to the use of a mood-altering chemical such as Valium, Librium, or marijuana. To others it appears that things are a little better. The appearance of control is the objective for the alcoholic, but it is obvious that the alcoholic is on something. Significant others know that the person is not normal, and most sense that this period of control is temporary and that the quality of life for the relapsing alcoholic is very shallow.

In this part of the catastrophe stage, many alcoholics begin and continue extensive drug use for years. They change course, further complicating the addiction, by using many new illegal drugs. It is here that some will experiment with cocaine for the first time and then go on to use it for a couple of years. Of course, the cocaine causes its own set of problems, and the person eventually must stop using it altogether. Whatever the drug the alcoholic turns to only produces another addiction and usually causes many more problems than the alcohol. Because it is illegal, the alcoholic, now addicted to cocaine or heroin or using LSD, PCP, or some other street drug, enters a new realm of dealers, pushers, and suppliers. Drug deals, big buys, and drug busts become a way of life. In a year or so, the drug addict no longer considers the problem to be alcohol. The drugs produce such devastating consequences, such as bad trips and jail, that alcohol seems a far lesser problem. But alcoholism is the root. The recovery from other drugs must encompass every area that alcoholism recovery covers.

In this stage of catastrophe, the alcoholic loses total control of drinking and of every area of life. The drinking can not be controlled by setting limits, changing the type of drink, abstinence without life-style changes, or using other drugs. Every attempt at control further damages the alcoholic and increases the problems of addiction. Each means used to try to make things better only makes the catastrophe worse and less bearable. Rather than making progress, the alcoholic gains more fears, apprehension, frustration, anxiety, irritability, and anger. The self-pity and dissatisfaction from the feelings of failure prevent him or her from seeing any hope or way out. With every form of treatment discontinued, and the alcoholic unwilling to ask for help, complete collapse becomes the only conclusion to the catastrophe stage.

If the alcoholic has broken off all contact with family or friends, he or she may binge alone for days until finally found by someone, or a physical illness forces hospitalization. More commonly, there are a lot of people around the relapsing alcoholic, each of them aware of the alcoholic's misery. Whether drinking or not, the person shows classic signs of depression, notably insomnia or long hours of continued sleeping. Overeating, undereating, or any radical change in eating habits point to the pain and agony being felt. Someone at this last stage of relapse appears both helpless and powerless. He or she is at a major crossroads. One road leads to ultimate recovery and the long-term sobriety everyone has wanted; it requires assistance by intervening significant others. The other road remaining in the helpless state—is more drinking, more depression, and more misery. The choice is usually determined by how those close to the alcoholic react throughout the relapse.

REACTIONS TO RELAPSE

Relapse is always discouraging, no matter what the problem. When the overeater returns to compulsive eating or the cancer patient in remission is found to have new cancer cells growing, it is very hard on everyone. In the case of alcoholism or drug addiction, it is doubly difficult because of the nature of the problem and the expectations of recovery. Because people associate relapse only with a return to chemicals, they are angry at the "choice" to use again. But if the people around the alcoholic could have known the full course of the progression, they might have prevented a return to the chemical by intervening long before the choice to use again was made. Consider the times when the relapse progression does end in drinking or using. How do people react, and how can those reactions be managed to help the person back toward recovery?

First of all, when someone drinks again, it is only normal that the family and friends become angry—they can't help it. They usually have such high hopes and dreams about a life free of alcohol and other drugs and want the best for the alcoholic. When things go wrong, there is tremendous disappointment and frustration, which surface as anger. It is not uncommon to feel that the alcoholic has betrayed everyone, that he or she had a responsibility to stay sober, no matter what, and that responsibility has been neglected. The spouse may believe that the alcoholic has once again chosen the bottle over the marriage. The anger that comes from all of these emotions is real and normal, but it must be managed appropriately or it will become destructive.

Anger must be expressed. If it is held in, it can turn either to bitter resentment or to uncontrollable rage. It can also make the bearer of the anger very ill, both emotionally and physically. But when it is expressed to the alcoholic in relapse, anger tends to drive a wedge between the family and the alcoholic. The alcoholic very likely feels tremendous guilt over the relapse, and the angry spouse or friend only magnifies the guilt and increases the isolation of the alcoholic. Because of these factors, one of the most important things for those close to the relapsed alcoholic is to summon help immediately. An experienced counselor can help with the resolution of the anger. Once it is expressed to the counselor, the bitterness is removed and no longer has the power to cut the relationship off. The counselor can help in looking at the situation as it exists and suggest the best plan of action to reverse the relapse. Someone overwhelmed with anger will not be able to form such a plan. The anger, if unresolved, will tend to turn the plan into a destructive rather than a constructive course of action.

In attempting to help someone out of relapse, it is extremely important not to revert to the old patterns that proved futile. Before recovery, the family often pleads, begs, threatens, and scolds in a desperate attempt to get the alcoholic to stop drinking. But the scolding and begging did not work before and are equally ineffective in reversing the relapse process. The best way to confront the alcoholic is in a calm, controlled, and consistent manner. Rather than bring up painful emotional events from the drinking past, the family member must stick to what has happened in relapse. It is best to describe the progression of relapse as it has occurred. The stages and symptoms in each stage should be pointed out one by one. Changes in the person should be noted. It should be pointed out how well he or she was doing. Positive actions that were being taken should be recalled and contrasted with recent negative changes. The downward spiral and the return to a depressive life-style should be presented in an unemotional and objective manner, yet convey the feelings of the person doing the presenting. That person should express how watching the changes has made him or her feel. A course of action or the next step should be recommended to the relapsing person. This is very similar to and in accordance with the intervention principles employed in initial recovery. The concerned other, whether spouse, child, or friend, is to state what happened, the feelings that resulted, and what action could be taken to change the progression. Through it all, hope for longterm recovery and sobriety is to be continually reinforced.

In addition to confronting the alcoholic in a supportive and directive manner, the family members need to examine how enabling is preventing the alcoholic from seeing the reality of the relapse. Just as threats and scolding are destructive to the alcoholic, all the enabling behaviors can allow the drinking to continue. Sometimes there is more motivation to cover up the drinking during relapse than before recovery was initiated. Before treatment, there is a good chance that fewer people knew about the drinking. Often the employer is unaware of a problem until involved in the aftercare planning process but, once involved, may watch the recovering alcoholic more closely than other employees. The spouse, knowing the employer is now aware of the problem, may attempt to cover up the drinking, giving the alcoholic permission to continue. No matter how painful the obvious consequences might be, the family must stop all enabling that promotes continued relapse.

Alanon attendance is also an important part of reversing the relapse. It also helps all of the family survive the potential trauma of a return to drinking. The support of the group can help the family maintain emotional strength and make the best decision for themselves and the alcoholic. Attendance at Alanon is important for another reason. It gives an undeniable message to the alcoholic that recovery is a priority and that the drinking remains a problem. If the alcoholic stops attending AA and the family continues to go to Alanon, the alcoholic is forced to think about why AA has been discontinued. While the alcoholic tries to convince everyone that drinking is not a problem, the family's Alanon attendance makes it clear that it is. There are many stories of alcoholics who were persuaded to stop drinking, not by words, but by the unwavering commitment of the family to go to Alanon.

Whatever the family does in the relapse process, they must not give up their efforts to help the alcoholic achieve long-term sobriety and recovery. It is easy to give up, but it helps no one. Many alcoholics relapse a few times and then go on to a meaningful and productive recovery. Hope needs to be reinforced in the alcoholic and in family members. The alcoholic has the ability to change, and with hope as a foundation, the family can act to initiate that change. Though in denial and functioning in a delusional world, the alcoholic has a choice to make. Every day of continued drinking is a negative decision. The family must do everything possible to support and reinforce a positive choice to change. This is especially important because the alcoholic's ability to choose is very limited due to denial and the use of mind-altering chemicals.

The family of the relapsed alcoholic must also accept recovery as a learning process. No one stops drinking and through treatment ''gets it.'' There is no instantaneous cure. A recovering alcoholic is one who never stops growing and learning. Relapse can be a time of learning, a time of coming face-to-face with limitations—ultimately, the beginning of a new commitment to protect oneself from relapse. The relapsed alcoholic may have been through a valuable time of testing the severity of the problem. Until the relapse, he or she may have not fully accepted the full degree of severity. There might have been a lack of understanding of just how important a system of protection is for long-term sobriety. If the relapse has taught the alcoholic these valuable and essential lessons, it can be the beginning of a realistic plan to obtain a lifetime of sobriety, one day at a time.

The beginning of long-term recovery and the end of relapse is a partnership effort. It is a partnership involving the alcoholic, the family, friends, employer, and others close to the alcoholic. The partnership is not brought about by people pointing fingers at each other and blaming; it happens because people care and take action based on the realistic hope that long-term sobriety can be accomplished. That partnership is also important in order to prevent the relapse from ever happening again. Everyone committed to the alcoholic staying sober must be committed to preventing relapse.

PREVENTING RELAPSE

The most important factor in preventing relapse is a well-balanced plan for recovery, as discussed in Chapter Eleven. Without a thorough recovery plan, sobriety is a temporary state. The more comprehensive the plan, the better the chances are for long-term recovery, and the more people involved in it, the better. The recovery plan should be so extensive that the physical, mental, emotional, social, and spiritual dimensions are all covered. The following is a short review of the vital components of a strong recovery plan:

- Attendance at aftercare meetings or some type of recovery support group
- Regular attendance at Alcoholics Anonymous, Narcotics Anonymous, Cocaine Anonymous, or some other self-help recovery support group
- Working the Twelve Steps of Alcoholics Anonymous
- Attendance by the family at Alanon and some AA meetings

- Attendance at lectures on alcoholism, drug addiction, recovery, and relapse
- Listening to tapes that reinforce a positive self-image by people who are recovering and experts in the field of chemical dependency
- Reading books about the disease concept of alcoholism, the family illness dimension of the problem, recovery, and relapse
- Regular exercise; the best is aerobic exercise activities that can involve the entire family
- Regular sleep habits that prevent late nights out
- A nutritious diet high in protein and complex carbohydrates while minimizing the intake of fats and sugars
- Regular utilization of relaxation techniques and meditation
- Continual analysis of relationships to determine the positive influences to develop and the negative influences to eliminate
- Changing activities from negative, high-pressure situations promoting drinking to more neutral settings that promote sobriety
- Developing a hobby such as cooking, painting, sculpture, or some craft that allows for creative expression
- Attendance at multifamily group therapy sessions where support, confrontation, interaction, and observations can reinforce the healing of the entire family
- Utilization of a highly experienced sponsor, counselor, and/or therapist to assist in the resolution of guilt, fear, and anger
- A search for ultimate truth and wisdom: discovering a life purpose by developing a relationship with God; continuing to turn over more of life to God and seeking God's direction and power for living

These components of a recovery plan offer the best chances for recovery. With the attitude of willingness to do whatever it takes, as many of these components as possible should be incorporated in the recovery plan. It is the best prevention against relapse.

There are some other important prevention measures that address relapse more specifically. One is a relapse plan of action. During treatment, the entire family should be taught the signs and symptoms of both relapse and recovery. The initial stages of relapse should be easily identifiable by the entire family. Actions that can reverse the relapse must be understood by everyone. A plan to be put in force at the first sign of relapse needs to be developed and agreed upon during the early stages of treatment.

A good relapse prevention plan will list the symptoms and the direct action to be taken. One symptom of relapse is discontinuing exercise and starting to eat foods very high in sugar. The relapse prevention plan might address this as follows:

Symptoms	Action Plan
Lack of exercise	1. Family will discuss it
Eating a lot of sugar	2. Talk to sponsor
	3. Discuss with counselor
	4. Increase AA attendance

This simple plan allows everyone to participate in the ongoing protection of the alcoholic. It provides specific action to be taken, action that is agreed upon in the early stages of treatment and recovery. Some would criticize this method, saying that it is the family working the alcoholic's program; others would say it is too restrictive. But these attitudes have contributed to a high relapse rate. Willingness to do whatever it takes means that, at times along the road to recovery, family and friends must be allowed to confront and redirect.

The best way for the alcoholic to avoid the ongoing intervention of family and friends in his or her recovery program is to have specific self-intervention plans written out and reviewed daily. A description of the steps toward relapse should be made by the alcoholic. Written in the first person, it should be an accurate portrayal of what is most likely to happen during relapse. This is not a plan for failure but a strong preventative measure. By personalizing the reality of relapse, the alcoholic can move more quickly to reverse the trend. Here is one alcoholic's beginning of such a description:

When I begin to relapse, I will most likely start lying to people around me. I'll find myself more and more trying to explain myself or cover up lies that I've even forgotten I told. I'll also start moving away from people who are supportive of me. I'll start thinking more about old drinking buddies and spend hours wondering how they are doing.

I'll probably stop exercising and taking care of myself

physically. My eating will return to a lot of sugar and a lot of chocolate. I'll probably gain some weight in the first weeks. . . .

The more detailed the description, the better. It is vital to identify indicators of complacency and compromising actions. It helps the alcoholic to avoid destructive mind games that prevent dealing with reality. The description of relapse is only the first step in the alcoholic's self-intervention. The second step is a plan of action to implement when relapse symptoms surface, such as this:

My Plan to Counteract Relapse
1. Call my sponsor to discuss my fears, attitudes, and actions.
2. Admit to my family that I am having problems and ask for help.
3. Phone my treatment counselor and arrange for an appointment to discuss my status and my problems.
4. If my counselor advises, I will return to treatment for a day or two to reinforce my sobriety.
5. Attend one AA meeting a day for at least thirty days.

If the symptoms are identified and personalized and a simple plan is developed to counter the symptoms, the alcoholic can change course before family and friends have to intervene. But that is not easy; the tendency is to cover up, hide, and distort reality. The alcoholic does not want to alarm the family or cause more problems. More than likely, the alcoholic is afraid of additional pressure or reprisals by the family. These fears must not be allowed to fuel relapse and delay recovery. The alcoholic must overcome the urge to withdraw at difficult times and instead reach for help just as he or she would if the problem were another illness like diabetes or even flu.

Self-intervention is always preferable when the symptoms of relapse begin to pile up. Initiating the plan as early as possible allows recovery to continue. If action is taken, the relapse symptoms will subside and the alcoholic's sobriety will stabilize again. Once the recovery plan is back in force and the alcoholic is more secure, a time of reflection and evaluation will enforce long-term sobriety. To prevent relapse again, all the threats to sobriety should be identified and resolved. The following chapter addresses these major threats to sobriety.

In summary, relapse is a progression that ultimately ends in a complete loss of control. It is a gradual process of moving further and further away from the recovery plan. The following are the four stages and the symptoms that exist within each stage.

1. *Complacency*: stopping those things that were designed to improve the quality of life
   - stopping going to AA or other recovery groups
   - stopping seeing a counselor
   - denial of need for a recovery plan
   - overconfidence: "I don't need to go to AA"
   - overinvolvement in helping others
   - denial of negative emotions such as fear
   - idleness
   - wishful thinking
   - lack of planning
   - daydreaming
   - living in a world of fantasy
   - unrealistic dreams
   - defensiveness about recovery
   - irresponsible life-style
   - self-analysis
   - brooding
   - intellectualization
   - belief that "I can handle it alone"
   - poor eating habits
   - lack of exercise
2. *Confusion*: doubting the real nature of the problem and the need for recovery
   - disconnected from support system
   - questioning if addiction was the real problem
   - questioning the need for abstinence, sobriety, counseling, or AA
   - difficulty with problem solving
   - increase in self-doubt
   - lowered self-esteem
   - doubt about disease concept of alcoholism
   - wondering if the alcoholic problem has been cured or conquered

- questioning the severity of the problem
- doubting that anyone can help
- more expectations turning into false hopes
- "there and then" living
- misperceptions about people, sobriety, and recovery
- irrational and inconsistent behavior

3. *Compromise*: returning to risky situations and risky people
   - needless exposure to high-pressure situations
   - easing back into drinking settings
   - returning to old playmates and playgrounds
   - expecting catering and pampering from others
   - further separation from support resources
   - increased anger and dissatisfaction
   - beginning of intense search for relief
   - obsession with thoughts of social drinking
   - conviction that one drink would not hurt
   - total lack of honesty
   - unwillingness to accept responsibility for problems
   - projecting blame on others
   - repeated use of "if only" statements—"If only my family understood me"
   - "I don't care" attitude
   - imposing sobriety on others
   - impulsive behavior
   - lack of daily structure
   - compensating behavior such as "workaholism"
   - deep apprehension about the future
   - hoarding of money
   - seeking over-the-counter relief

4. *Catastrophe*: collapse of the ability to maintain control
   - use of prescription mood-altering drugs
   - experimentation with other mood-altering and addicting drugs
   - return to the chemical of choice
   - attempts to limit consumption
   - long binges
   - complete loss of control
   - physical exhaustion
   - emotional collapse
   - severe depression
   - psychotic break

- severe illness
- divorce
- suicide attempts
- radical changes in eating and sleeping habits
- appearance of helplessness or powerlessness

It is important to remember that relapse is a part of the disease and of recovery from alcoholism. It is a time of great disappointment and negative emotions, but it is also a time to come face-to-face with the reality of recovery and a society that is not supportive of recovery. Relapse can be the beginning of a realistic recovery process that leads to a better quality of life and peace with the world. Although it is a part of recovery, relapse can be prevented. To prevent it, the alcoholic must be willing to do whatever it takes. Whatever it takes means eliminating everything that is a threat to the precious condition of sobriety.

CHAPTER THIRTEEN

TEN MAJOR THREATS TO SOBRIETY

For recovering alcoholics, sobriety becomes the major priority of life. No thing, place, or person must be allowed to interfere with the ability to live one day at a time without alcohol or other drugs. On top of that abstinence, the building of a meaningful life must not be blocked for any reason. To ensure that sobriety is maintained, it is necessary to be familiar with the major threats to sobriety that are experienced by most recovering alcoholics. Once aware of the threats, alcoholics can plan appropriately to eliminate these dangerous trigger points of relapse.

For years, Alcoholics Anonymous has recognized four major threats to sobriety. These threats are mentioned frequently in the form of an acronym, the word HALT: *H*ungry, *A*ngry, *L*onely, and *T*ired. Alcoholics frequently admonish each other to not become too hungry, angry, lonely, or tired, because it is in these four states that people often drink again or begin the relapse process toward drinking. This simple word has helped thousands of people maintain sobriety because they were aware of the dangers of these four conditions. These are not the only threats that lead alcoholics out of recovery and into relapse. These four have been expanded and developed into ten major threats.

The ten major threats to sobriety are perhaps the most important ten pieces of information for recovering alcoholics to know. If alcoholics will learn of these threats and avoid them, a sobriety of high quality can be preserved. Recognizing them is just the first step; sobriety is preserved only when a recovery plan is developed that will avoid these ten problems.

THREAT NUMBER ONE: GUILT

There is a story about an elephant and an ant that illustrates the effect of guilt on many alcoholics, both in relapse and recovery. An elephant and an ant both went off to college to pursue an education. They ended up at the same college with exactly the same major, zoology. Although to most, these two had little in common, they grew to like each other very much. In fact, they fell in love. Both family and friends tried to point out the extreme differences between the two. They tried to explain the magnitude of the problems each would face. No one felt that either an elephant or an ant should marry outside of his or her phylum. But these two could not be stopped; they were beyond reasoning. So it was that this very large elephant and this very small ant decided to marry. And marry they did.

On the honeymoon night it was a wonderful time for both the elephant and the ant. Their first night of marriage was more fun than either had ever expected. It seemed that they were proving the critics wrong.

The next morning, after a fantastic night, the ant awoke to a terrible tragedy. The poor elephant was dead. The little ant, in shock and greatly depressed, looked up to God and moaned: "Just my luck! One night of pleasure, and I spend the rest of my life digging a grave."

Of course, it's a dumb little story, but it illustrates a drastic mistake made by many recovering alcoholics. They think that their life will be filled with hard labor to cover their past misdeeds. Rather than living life to the fullest, they simply destroy themselves and dig their own graves. They do not feel worthy of a victorious and productive life. They settle for second and third best, living in misery without alcohol and without anything else, all because of unresolved feelings of guilt.

I was down in Mason, Texas, back in January of 1986 with about 350 of the town's 2,000 residents. The occasion was the dedication of a new alcoholism treatment program called Intercept at Mason Memorial Hospital. The new director of the program went to the podium to address the crowd and explain the concepts behind this new alcohol treatment center. In describing to the Mason residents what the people would be like, he used this phrase: "These are not bad people who need to be good, these are sick people who need to get well." This one attitude is probably the most important attitude for sustaining long-term sobriety.

The stigma of alcoholism has led many to label themselves as bad or immoral. These labels result in extreme feelings of guilt. Alcoholics trying to recover with this heavy burden of guilt often fail to find happiness. Until the guilt is resolved, a miserable existence is about all that can be expected for the alcoholic. I believe that more alcoholics relapse because of unresolved guilt than for any other reason. It is by far the worst plague in the alcoholic's recovery. Unless it is resolved, it is the most dangerous threat to sobriety.

The reason for the guilt is that the alcoholics have refused to accept, or simply do not know, that alcoholism is a disease. Instead, they continue to believe that the alcoholism is a result of an emotional weakness, immorality, or direct punishment from God. They do not accept that alcoholism is a disease that means a person cannot drink. Instead they see themselves as second-class citizens, as underprivileged misfits who no longer belong. They feel terrible about themselves, what they did while they were drinking, and their future as alcoholics.

Alcoholics must be able to accept themselves as sick people who need to get well. They must totally buy into the disease concept of alcoholism. They must accept that the difference from others is a physiological one, not one of integrity, moral fiber, or strength. If alcoholics see it any other way, their recovery path will lead only to more disappointment. They will try to become better, to be good, or they will attempt to grow stronger. No amount of goodness or strength will change the inability to drink and process alcohol like other people; the goal must be acceptance of that basic premise of alcoholism. If it is not accepted, guilt will increase, because no one can become good enough or strong enough to overcome alcoholism. As people repeatedly try and fail, they feel greater guilt about having the problem. They constantly feel a growing ache inside. That ache is a needless feeling of being a bad person who must become good.

The reality is that no one is perfect. No one goes through life without causing some sort of problem or hurting some people. The beauty of recovery is the ability to start over every day, to accept that a mistake has been made or someone has been hurt, and make amends for it. The guilt trip taken by many alcoholics makes admitting mistakes more difficult. Trying to reach an unattainable goal of perfection, the alcoholic refuses to admit weaknesses that even the strongest possess. This only complicates recovery and prevents growth and maturity in relationships.

Treatment for alcoholism must help alcoholics let go of the past and the feelings associated with it. Crying, weeping, moaning, wailing, gnashing of teeth, or any form of self-inflicted pain will not change the past. They only prevent people from living in the present and achieving a desirable future. So many alcoholics pass up a new life because of constantly reliving the old life, which cannot be changed. The old life must be let go; it must be traded in for new opportunities and new areas of growth free of guilt and remorse.

In the book *Hooked on Life*, by Tim Timmons and Stephen Arterburn, there is a presentation on the need to let go of the past. The book discusses people who live their lives through the rearview mirror that reveals only the past. For many, that rearview mirror is larger than today's reality. They study and relive each mistake of the rearview past and finally repeat the past in future forms of failure. It is a sad and wasteful way of life, but one that is practiced by many.

Alcoholics must shrink their rearview mirrors of the past. They must shrink them so that life, the life of today and tomorrow, can be experienced. One very successful way to shrink the past and the guilt found there is by making amends. Freedom from the past has been found by many who have taken the time to write down on paper who has been hurt by the drinking, then, where it would not cause further harm, set out to make amends for past hurts. (These are the eighth and ninth steps of the Alcoholics Anonymous program.) It is not an easy task. It requires strength and courage, but painful as it is, it is nothing compared to the pain of a lifetime of living in an unchangeable past.

Making amends can be accomplished in many ways. It can be done by repaying some money that was borrowed or stolen, or admitting to a lie; more often than not, it can be done with a simple phone call. Acknowledging what happened and asking for forgiveness can constitute amends in most instances. It is all that it takes to break the bonds of guilt and experience emotional freedom. It is astounding how the burden of guilt lightens with every person who is contacted. When all is done, the alcoholic can look anyone in the eye with nothing to hide.

Guilt is so destructive because it separates people from each other and keeps them apart. The strands of a relationship can only be strengthened when communication occurs. Guilt forms a barrier between people. It destroys the ability to communicate openly. The end result is isolation and alienation. Alcoholics cannot recover in isolation; they need support from others. Amends must be made and guilt must be resolved if alcoholics are to reenter supportive relationships that enhance sobriety.

Making amends has another powerful impact on the problem of guilt. It allows alcoholics to hear from others that they are forgiven. When others tell alcoholics that they no longer hold a grudge, that forgiveness is complete; alcoholics can forgive themselves, and it is important for them to do this. The self-condemnation that flourished during drinking must be replaced with self-forgiveness. Two requisites for life without guilt are accepting alcoholism as a disease and making amends for past mistakes. When these are completed, alcoholics' attitudes change dramatically. They are able to accept sobriety as a gift and feel deserving of a new life.

There is one last key to resolving the threat of guilt. It is attending to the spiritual dimension of recovery. Spirituality must not be ignored but must be developed, just as any other area of recovery. It is the one area of recovery that brings ultimate forgiveness for the guilt from the past. As someone searches for truth, the end of that search is reached at the knowledge of God, a God who created everyone, problems and all. The realization that a Supreme Being made us, and knew the problems we would cause before we ever caused them, is very important. To know of the special provision God made for our forgiveness is even more important. Accepting God's forgiveness allows self-forgiveness and freedom from guilt. This is found only when a person searches for God's truth and then, from that truth, grows spiritually.

To recover, life must be lived one day at a time. Nothing must divert the alcoholic from living in the present. Guilt binds the alcoholic to the past and produces isolation and alienation in the present. It must be resolved if supportive relationships are to grow and mature. The pain and agony of guilt can be very intense. Many alcoholics have returned to drinking because the guilt is so strong and the pain so deep. They have sought instant relief and, instead of easing the pain, have deepened their wounds. This threat can be reversed through making amends, open confession, and accepting forgiveness from God.

THREAT NUMBER TWO:
UNHEALTHY RELATIONSHIPS

Unhealthy relationships can lure an alcoholic out of recovery and into relapse. They can obscure the alcoholic's view of reality and destroy a person's plan of recovery. In the initial stages of recovery, relationships must be analyzed for their potential impact on recovery. With the help of sponsors, counselors, and other support personnel, negative relationships can be developed into positive forces for recovery. Until that is accomplished, they can be a major threat to recovery.

At times, alcoholics will naïvely start recovery with the belief that everyone is pulling for them and will be supportive of recovery. They trust the motives of family, friends, and fellow employees. This can be a tragic mistake. Alcoholics must accept that their sobriety causes problems for some people who have grown dependent on their being drunk. This is not a very popular area to get into, but it is vital for alcoholics to know the reality of sabotage that sometimes exists among the alcoholic's relationships.

Sabotage of recovery is not usually an overt act. Those involved are often unconscious that they are being destructive, but the fact remains that there are individuals who will benefit from a return to drinking. For example, old drinking buddies who have drinking problems of their own may feel threatened by the recovering alcoholic's abstinence. Recovery by a close friend forces the practicing alcoholic to face the reality of his or her own drinking problem. It certainly produces an uncomfortable feeling when an old friend says no to a drink while the drinking buddy orders the twelfth drink of the evening. This problem drinker or alcoholic is not likely to be thrilled over the recovering alcoholic's decision to not drink. From that discomfort may come some strong urgings to have "just one drink." The recovering alcoholic needs to be prepared for that kind of pressure and be ready to react quickly. The best reaction is to leave that person immediately and not return to his or her company for a long time.

There are other problems that can arise at the workplace. For years a subordinate or a peer may have been watching the alcoholic's performance deteriorate and speculating about the approaching wreck of the alcoholic's career. This coworker may have a definite dream or plan to fill the position once the alcoholic is fired. Additionally, the alcoholic's worsening performance may place a coworker's performance in a more positive light.

The recovery of the alcoholic destroys the opportunity for someone to advance in his or her place. It also can make the performance of other workers appear unacceptable; the recovering alcoholic returning to work is often more motivated to produce than coworkers. The boss, astonished at the complete turnaround in performance and attitude, may lavish praise on the recovering alcoholic. This can produce jealousy from other employees, who may nudge the alcoholic toward a return to drinking. Subtle hints and frequent exposure to drinking situations may be used to lure the alcoholic back to the bottle. The alcoholic must not assume that everyone at work is supportive of his or her sobriety and must be aware of the possible negative reinforcement from fellow workers.

There are those closer to the alcoholic than fellow employees who may gain from a return to drinking by the alcoholic. These are family members who have not adjusted to new roles while the alcoholic has been learning to let go of the role of the drunk. A spouse may have spent a lifetime with the alcoholic and putting up with all the problems associated with drinking. This person may be classified as a "saint" or a "martyr" to those who have watched the years of patient handling of the alcoholic. Once recovering, the alcoholic becomes the focus of attention; praise once given the spouse is directed at the alcoholic who has made such a tremendous change. The "saint," feeling loss of "sainthood," may unconsciously lead the alcoholic back into drinking. This might be done by suggesting that since everything is so great and the alcoholic has done so well, a drink is a just reward. It may sound bizarre and illogical, but it happens all the time. You may remember just such an incident from Chapter Six.

A female alcoholic married to a very insecure man must be

extremely careful about her spouse's motives. A weak man may feel dominant and in control while his wife is drinking abusively. He may feel superior in the relationship because of his wife's inability to stop drinking; he may see her as unable to threaten his virility. Once the female begins recovery, the weak male may feel threatened for his life. He may fear her dominance or even abandonment once she discovers his faults and weaknesses. He may wonder if she will look to a greater, stronger companion now that the drinking is over. Consequently, he may sabotage the wife's recovery. To regain his feelings of superiority, he may do everything in his power to push her back into the role of sick drinker. He may threaten, batter, or rebuke in an attempt to get his wife to drink again. These bizarre relationships exist when the family goes untreated. They are remedied when identified and resolved so that everyone can move into healthier roles that do not depend on or benefit from the alcoholic's return to drinking.

To ward off effectively the threats to sobriety from unhealthy relationships, alcoholics need to ask some very difficult questions. Painful as it may be, each alcoholic needs to ask, "Who in my life would benefit from my being drunk again?" And in the uncomfortable times of recovery, the alcoholic must stop to consider, "Who in my life is subtly pushing me toward relapse?" There are those who harbor thinly disguised contempt for the remarkable change that comes in the life of the recovering alcoholic. These people must be identified and avoided, especially early in the recovery process. By identifying the unhealthy motives in unsupportive relationships, a subtle seduction into relapse can be avoided.

There is another type of highly destructive threat to sobriety from relationships. This stems from relationships that develop early in recovery. Falling in love early in the treatment process usually leads to disaster. It removes the focus from recovery and onto another person. A dependency on alcohol and drugs can be converted to a dependency on another person. No matter how genuine the motives may appear, the foundation of the relationship is an attempt to find relief.

It is common to see people who are cross-addicted to two or more chemicals; alcoholics are often addicted to Valium or some other drug. When relief through alcohol is not convenient or available, relief is achieved through another substance. The cross-addiction does not have to involve another chemical. It can be a sexual addiction that replaces the focus on recovery from alcoholism. The alcoholic, seeking relief and euphoria, may search out repeated sexual involvement to escape. These repeated unhealthy relationships distort reality and stop recovery. They must be avoided at all costs.

There are many examples of how early romantic and/or sexual involvement has resulted in a derailed recovery. One such case involved a woman who had become addicted to prescription painkillers in postoperative treatment following extensive surgery. She entered treatment to rid herself of the addiction, but in the midst of the treatment process, she fell in love with a singer. He was a true romantic, a fulfillment of her dreams of breaking out of her role as a middle-class housewife. They both felt that their love was real, and pursued each other after they were discharged. She left her husband to move into the singer's apartment. Having her as a goal, he was highly motivated to maintain his sobriety. She thought he had it all together and hoped that a new life was in store for both of them, but her hopes were short-lived. Just when everything was going well, he began to drink again.

This woman had never known her singer when he was drinking. It was a part of him that she thought was gone forever. But she was devastated as his drinking threw him into fits of rage and uncontrollable violence. Finally, when he had drunk himself into a half-stupor, she persuaded him to go back to the hospital with her. She loaded him into the car and took off. On the way he threw up repeatedly on her and her clean car. He burned cigarette holes all over her seats. When she arrived at the hospital, she was terrified. I went to the car to help him inside; the stench of vomit and booze was sickening. It was a distant world from the fantasy she had had of life with a romantic singer.

Of course she returned to her drugs, and he, embarrassed and hurt, left treatment after only one day. Two people once full of great potential became two destructive partners who destroyed each other's hopes. It began with a sexual attraction fueled by a sexual encounter in the early stages of treatment. For recovery to be real, alcoholics must stop drinking. They must stop using alcohol and drugs, but they must also stop using sex and relationships and people. They must avoid the threat that an unhealthy relationship can have on the state of sobriety. They must be especially careful to avoid sexual relationships that appear to promise relief and end up providing guilt, pain, and emptiness. Alcoholics Anonymous suggests strongly that no important decisions be made during the first year of sobriety and is particularly firm on the undesirability of establishing a romantic relationship.

The last threat to sobriety in the area of relationships is often neglected. Rather than sabotaging or engaging in a sexual relationship, it is loneliness, where no relationships exist at all. Relationships are not easy to develop, but they are essential for recovery. Recovery cannot happen in a vacuum devoid of growing, maturing relationships. The threat of loneliness must be countered by seeking out opportunities to develop healthy relationships. AA meetings, PTA, church, choir, the symphony are all places where relationships can be formed. Often alcoholics fail to achieve sobriety because they convince themselves that they are different. They want to believe that they need to be alone and free from the demands of relationships. That attitude is very unhealthy; recovery must encompass rebuilding old relationships and developing new and healthy ones. Without the effort, sobriety and recovery are greatly threatened.

This threat of unhealthy relationships must be defeated through the process of social recovery. Changing "playmates and playgrounds" from the drinking days must be a priority. New, healthy relationships, supportive of recovery, must replace old relationships that existed only through the common bond of the bottle. Both family and friends must adjust and grow, even change roles so that the alcoholic is not lured back into drinking. When all the relationships of the alcoholic are supportive of the changes brought about through recovery, relapse is prevented and recovery is preserved.

THREAT NUMBER THREE: HOLIDAYS

When Thanksgiving, Christmas, and New Year's approach, the alcoholic must be prepared to add extra means of protection from relapse. These holidays and the emotions and activities that surround them are a major threat to recovery. They must not be taken for granted or ignored. The relapse rate is very high during and shortly after these occasions because alcoholics do not realize the impact that they can have on recovery. Often alcoholics end the holidays depressed and anxious, with bills that cannot be paid and expectations that cannot be met.

One of the principal relapse factors involving the holidays is unrealistic expectations that go unfulfilled. There is danger in expecting too much from times with the family. Often alcoholics will fantasize about how wonderful a first sober Christmas will be. They may fantasize about a warm and loving time with the family. What actually happens is a major disappointment. Rather than warm feelings of affection, often great tension keeps everyone on edge. Old resentments may surface, and feelings of anger, pent up for years, are openly expressed. The hoped-for dream of family warmth turns into a nightmare of dissension and disillusionment. The unprepared alcoholic may find the time so painful that he or she drinks again.

The alcoholic will often expect too much from family and friends not seen since the previous holiday season. The recovering alcoholic often changes radically and is caught up in the process of growing and may mistakenly believe that everyone else is also experiencing great change and growth. It is a huge disappointment to discover that others have not changed, that they are holding on to old behaviors and old attitudes. Some of those old attitudes are directed at the recovering alcoholic. As the alcoholic feels the anger, hurt, or bitterness that some still harbor over things that happened years ago, the urge to escape may intensify. Commonly, the feeling of "What's the use?" creeps in, and the alcoholic moves toward drinking rather than preserving sobriety.

The alcoholic must develop realistic expectations about the holidays. There must not be a false hope that everyone is going to forget and forgive the alcoholic for past holidays that might have been ruined by drinking. People need time to resolve those feelings. It may take several holidays before trust is reestablished. The alcoholic must call upon support resources that can help through difficult times with family and friends. Eventually it will get better, but the alcoholic who expects to be treated like a hero because of one holiday without alcohol will probably be very dissatisfied with others' reactions.

One final comment on the holidays: they are extremely dangerous to another group of alcoholics, those who no longer have families. Their loneliness often intensifies around the holidays. It seems that unresolved guilt emerges with greater force as the alcoholic wishes to have what others appear to be enjoying. The holidays are a terrible time to be alone. The best way to combat the problem is to plan ahead. The alcoholic may need to open up at an AA meeting and ask for help through the holiday season. Or better yet, he or she may invite others over who would probably spend the holidays alone. Anything to keep busy and active with people is better than sitting at home alone, brooding over times that never were and fantasy Christmases that never will be. The holidays are difficult for many people, both alcoholic and nonalcoholic alike. Whether the family is involved or not, the alcoholic must plan to have extra support around those times and think realistically about what is to be expected from family and friends. The holidays are times of heavier drinking and more occasions to drink. Pressure to drink, plus emotional pain from the family, can prove to be too much for the unprepared alcoholic.

THREAT NUMBER FOUR: HUNGER

Under the threat of hunger come all of the recovery problems associated with eating. Eating correctly can make recovery much more stable and easily managed. But many alcoholics ignore this area of physical recovery. They fail to see the connection between sugar and alcohol. They do not fully understand how valuable the proper food can be in controlling the urge to drink.

One of the things that happens in addiction to alcohol is the development of the *urge* to drink. This could be called an obsession with alcohol or the compulsion to drink. For alcoholics, this urge is very real. It can completely take over the person's thought processes and destroy any ability to concentrate. The urge to drink must be satisfied. Of course, the urge is not a mere manifestation of the mind. It is a result of the addiction of the body. It comes from the cells craving the substance that they have adjusted to. For the practicing alcoholic, it is alcohol that eases the urge and allows the mind to focus on other things.

The body, once addicted to alcohol, has a difficult time differentiating between the source of urges. This is why hunger can be so detrimental to sobriety. The hungry person may feel the urge to eat, but the mind, so used to the old urge to drink, may not interpret the hunger urge for what it is. The mind may become convinced that the only way to satisfy the urge is to have another drink. Now, whether or not the person drinks again, this is a very difficult state of mind to manage, and, for the most part, it is avoidable.

Probably the biggest culprit in developing intense hunger urges is sugar. Ingestion of high levels of sugar produces greater hunger pangs and urges that need to be satisfied. As the blood sugar level increases through eating foods full of sugar, the alcoholic experiences a satisfying "sugar high." It is a dangerous condition. The blood sugar level drops suddenly and leaves the alcoholic depressed, sluggish, and craving sugar. The craving and urge for sugar is often satisfied by a return to drinking. In talking to hundreds of alcoholics who have relapsed, and discussing the events leading up to a return to drinking, a similar story is often told: the alcoholic starts to binge on foods high in sugar content. Ice cream, candy, pies, cakes, and other junk foods precede the return to alcohol for many alcoholics. Protection from relapse must include avoidance of foods high in sugar and awareness of the danger of sugar binges.

Food can be used as a mood stabilizer in recovery. Foods high in protein and in complex carbohydrates, free of sugar, allow moods to stabilize. Extreme emotional highs and lows from rapidly changing blood sugar levels can be avoided with nutritious foods. The temptation to get a quick lift from sugar must be avoided at all costs. Some alcoholics use a line of Dorothy Parker's as a slogan: "Candy is dandy, but liquor is quicker." This adage summarizes the danger in using high-sugar foods. Sugar produces a pleasant effect, an initial mood change, but it is only temporary. Failing to achieve desired results from sugar or candy, many alcoholics move back into their drug of choice, alcohol. A high level of sugar ingestion must be seen for what it is, one step away from a return to alcohol, and avoided at all costs. About the only significant flaw to be found in AA is its widespread practice of serving unlimited cakes, doughnuts, and cookies along with coffee at most meetings, and recommendations, particularly from older members, that cravings for drink be fought off with high-sugar foods. AA thinking on this matter was established before modern nutritional knowledge developed, and this view is a counterproductive relic of the past. Nutritionally aware new members are making some inroads in this area.

THREAT NUMBER FIVE: HIGH-PRESSURE SITUATIONS

An important maxim for recovery is "Never stay too long where you do not belong." Remaining in a high-pressure situation can wear down one's resistance, minute by minute, until the will to preserve sobriety is gone. High-pressure situations can have the same effect as the Chinese water torture. A person's strength is worn down until there is a final break or collapse. To avoid losing the will to recover, high-pressure situations must be identified and avoided. The alcoholic must realize that resistance to stress is lowest in the early days of recovery. Until the central nervous system heals, stress and pressure are highly destructive for the alcoholic.

High-pressure situations exist where conflict continues between two people. If the boss is one who belittles and berates day after day, a new job should be sought. No one should be subjected to daily criticism and unnecessary pressure early in recovery. A certain coworker may be a source of constant conflict; if there is someone who makes the alcoholic dread going to work in the morning, perhaps a transfer can be made to a more comfortable setting. If work is a place of high pressure and intense conflict, it can be the trigger for relapse. Change, though difficult or painful, must be made if recovery is to be maintained.

Often the most intense pressure and conflict occur in the home of the recovering alcoholic. As everyone tries to adjust and searches for new roles, the pressure can be great. Emotions do not heal quickly. Bitterness will often remain and infect even the most insignificant conversations. If the pressure is too high, the alcoholic must seek an alternative until the home can become a more supportive environment. The best alternative, when available, is a halfway house and a family therapist. The halfway house provides a supportive living space while the family heals under the care of a trained family therapist. Years of family problems cannot be expected to vanish in a day or four weeks or even a year. When the problems are acute, assistance is needed to motivate the whole family toward recovery while the alcoholic establishes a stable sobriety.

Other high-pressure situations that threaten sobriety involve settings where alcohol and heavy drinking are standard. This setting could be a work environment where there is a large percentage of heavy drinkers, where abstainers may be frowned upon and considered "wimpy." That is no place for a newly recovered alcoholic to establish sobriety. Family gatherings or reunions where almost everyone gets drunk are not the healthiest places to spend time. Frequently patronizing bars and old drinking hangouts can be dangerously seductive for the alcoholic. The unconscious desire to be part of the crowd can provide enough internal pressure to trigger a relapse.

Every alcoholic will benefit from thoroughly analyzing work, play, and family situations to identify high-pressure threats to sobriety. Negative environments must be eliminated. They should be replaced with positive, supportive people and settings that encourage recovery. When the alcoholic finds himself or herself in a very intense high-pressure situation, the most valuable skill for ongoing sobriety is knowing how to walk away from the temptation. No event, gathering, or establishment is more important than sobriety. Learning to leave those places behind and to replace them with healthy settings is essential for a high-quality life-style without alcohol.

THREAT NUMBER SIX: ANGER

Those who live with an alcoholic are all too familiar with the anger that intensifies over the years of drinking. Some even believe anger is the main problem for the alcoholic, that the alcoholic's uncontrollable anger is the central reason for drinking, and that if the anger is resolved, the need to drink will no longer exist. The theory, of course, has it backward: the anger is caused by the high alcohol consumption.

The connection between alcohol and anger is discussed elsewhere, but it is worthwhile to go over some of it in this context. As the alcohol saturates the alcoholic's body, it produces toxic and irritating effects on the central nervous system. As the drinking continues, the emotional barometer elevates, and the alcoholic moves into anger and fits of rage. The physiological basis for this is either a body irritated from the large amounts of alcohol or a body withdrawing from the alcohol. There is also a psychological basis for the anger. As the alcoholic hears how he or she should be able to control the problem, and as there is a growing awareness that the ability to control the drinking is weakening, the alcoholic becomes angrier at himself or herself. The more times the alcoholic fails at stopping drinking, the greater the anger.

Treatment does not immediately take care of this aspect of emotional recovery. It requires a lot of time. It also requires a lot of forgiveness. After stopping drinking, the alcoholic may be angry at the prospect of a life without alcohol. He or she may be directly angry at God for the problem of alcoholism. The answer? Forgive God. Forgive God for not making a perfect world without frustration. Forgive God for not meeting everyone's expectations. That forgiveness must be offered to other people, too. If the alcoholic can forgive family and friends, anger dies. The alcoholic must also forgive himself or herself. Self-hatred and self-anger destroy the ability to remain sober. They must be eliminated from the alcoholic's thoughts and feelings. This is best done with the help of an experienced therapist. The therapist can lead the alcoholic toward forgiving God, others, self, and the world.

Anger frequently is found in people who are expecting too much from others. Their unrealistic expectations, when unmet, produce anger and frustration. The alcoholic may also expect too much too soon from recovery, and every time a struggle or difficulty requires some pain and discomfort, the anger may go out of control. The alcoholic must expect difficult times in the maturing process rather than instant change and ease. This is a realistic acceptance of the condition. Acceptance of the disease, the problems, and the nature of life heals the alcoholic's anger, and is a goal to strive for. In the state of acceptance there is much comfort and serenity. But acceptance will not be contained within the mind and spirit of an angry person. If acceptance is to grow, anger must be pushed out. The primary step in moving from anger to acceptance is putting forth the effort to forgive. Offering forgiveness to others is the beginning of accepting them the way they are. Offering forgiveness for oneself is the beginning of self-acceptance.

When acceptance and forgiveness are not established as goals, anger will hamper the recovery process, progressing and intensifying until it reaches the state of uncontrollable rage. It is a pattern that is experienced by many alcoholics. When a person is unforgiving and living with unrealistic expectations, there are all sorts of major and minor irritations. People's voices grate, and people's silence becomes irritating. It is irritating to stay at home and irritating to be away. The irritations add up, building on top of one another until the state of anger is produced.

IRRITATION → ANGER

If the anger is not resolved through acceptance and forgiveness, it develops into hatred. This is self-hatred, which is the most intense. Then there is hatred for others and hatred for God. No attempt to hide this hatred can mask its existence. It becomes obvious. People start to say, "Now, there goes an angry person," or "Hate is written all over that face." The person full of hatred is depressed and angry. Nothing satisfies and everything disappoints.

IRRITATION → ANGER → HATRED

Hate soon turns into a life of bitterness. The bitter individual is full of all sorts of illogical and grossly inappropriate resentments. The bitterness affects every relationship by destroying any hope of any positive feelings for another. Movies portray the cranky old man who is bitter at life and everyone living; he resents anyone having a good time or trying to help him enjoy life. There are a lot of cranky old men and women not over thirty or forty years old. To them, the entire world is at fault. It is the *world* that is wrong—its people and everything they do. Bitterness is not a cheerful companion, but some refuse to replace it with forgiveness and acceptance.

Alcoholics Anonymous places considerable emphasis on the importance of giving up past resentments and not creating new ones. Through the support of other alcoholics and working the twelve steps, the recovering person learns to resolve resentments by "letting go." Vengeance and getting even is left to God. Correcting people or transforming them into "better" people is left to God. With that approach to resentment, the emotional load remains light and under control. Bitterness is not given a foothold. It is dissolved before it starts.

IRRITATION → ANGER → HATRED → BITTERNESS

At any point along the way from momentary irritation to a life-style of bitterness, the alcoholic may reach complete lack of control and move into a state of rage.

IRRITATION—ANGER—HATRED—BITTERNESS

RAGE

Acting out of rage, the alcoholic is completely out of control. The behavior directly parallels drinking days when family discussions quickly escalated into family violence. When this point is reached, it is too late. Whatever happens will probably cause more feelings of guilt and remorse. Relapse will be in full force.

Anger must be controlled and resolved before it becomes hatred, bitterness, or especially rage. The alcoholic must no longer have unrealistic expectations that cause anger as each one goes unmet. The solution is forgiveness and acceptance. Since it is hard to accomplish that alone, it is helpful to obtain assistance from a sponsor if one is in AA, a friend, or a counselor—someone who can be a reminder to stop trying to run the world and *accept* the way God wants it run. When the alcoholic allows God to be in control and manage the world, especially the alcoholic's world, there is nothing to be angry about. There are no irritations or dissatisfactions. Reassurance and acceptance are felt, even when encountering the toughest of problems. It becomes a way of life and a preserver of sobriety.

THREAT NUMBER SEVEN: LACK OF SLEEP

When I first began working with alcoholics back in Fort Worth, I met a lady who clued me in to this major problem in recovery. She was convinced that alcoholic relapse was most often precipitated by the inability to sleep. She placed insomnia and sleep irregularities at the top of the list of threats to sobriety. She would continually remind those in the alcoholism field that restful sleep must be a priority in recovery. Any alcoholic who cannot find adequate rest is a prime candidate for relapse.

A phenomenal number of alcoholics have great difficulty with sleep. Their early days of recovery find them tired and sluggish. A very tired alcoholic is a very fragile alcoholic. Any alcoholic who has problems finding rest should not accept it as a permanent condition. There are things that can be done to correct the problem. Although abnormal sleep *is* normal in the very earliest days of recovery, there are ways for the alcoholic to consistently find rest and the ability to sleep.

First of all, sleep problems are normal right after stopping the alcohol and drugs; nights are commonly filled with restlessness, tossing, and turning. The alcoholic awakens feeling more tired than when he or she went to bed. Nightmares may interrupt sleep, or disquieting dreams may be experienced night after night. Many of these sleep problems are a result of the central nervous system adjusting to a chemical-free existence. The nervous system has been damaged from being saturated by the alcohol or in withdrawal from it, and while the nerves are healing, rest is frequently interrupted and sleep cannot be attained. These problems are intensified in individuals who do not act in ways that will minimize sleep disturbances.

There are ways to correct sleep problems. Special sleep disorder units have been set up across the country. Sometimes surgery is required to allow continued breathing; in some people, breathing stops, and the alcoholic is repeatedly jolted awake when it begins again. Many alcoholics have received their first full night's sleep after having the minor surgery. Anyone who is always suffering from sleep deprivation should consult a physician about the possible need to utilize one of these sleep disorder clinics. It can completely change a person's life; many alcoholics can attest to phenomenal results in a very short time.

There are less drastic means used to correct many sleep problems. They work for alcoholics and nonalcoholics alike. The first area that needs to be explored is the psychological one. Depression can be a cause of sleep problems; so can excess stress that is not worked off. A wide range of emotional problems, from fear to low self-esteem, may promote inability to find rest. Working with a counselor to resolve these problems may provide the needed relief.

Closely allied to the psychological dimension are mental techniques that produce rest. Memorization of poetry and Scripture have been used to create a deep sleep state. The insomniac takes the poem or Scripture passage to bed and reads it until it is learned by heart. Then the light is turned out, and the passage is repeated over and over. The Twenty-third Psalm is a favorite of many who need help sleeping. Focusing on the words and the images within the passage blocks the stresses and stimuli from the outside world. Some take the principle even further and meditate on great truths. They become engulfed in words and meanings and fall comfortably asleep in the middle of the meditation. This method of correcting sleep problems can add depth and meaning to life while it allows rest.

The mind can rest much easier with the help of the body. The basic concepts of physical recovery are helpful in turning around a sleep disorder. Often the answer is very simple. Someone who never exercises will be more tense than someone who makes exercise a part of a daily routine. Or is it any wonder that someone who drinks about twenty cups of coffee a day, with over thirteen hundred milligrams of caffeine, has a hard time sleeping at night? I do not think so. Nor is it hard to accept that consuming two six-packs of caffeinated colas will produce a sleep problem. Some people are more sensitive to caffeine than others and cannot find adequate rest if they drink even one cola or one cup of coffee after three in the afternoon. Any alcoholic finding it hard to sleep should do without all caffeine for at least a month, which will allow enough time for the body to adjust to the lack of daily stimulation. This may prove to be a very simple cure to a very difficult problem.

Nutrition can play a vital role in getting good rest. Nutritionists say that it is best to eat heavier early in the day and lighter toward the end of the day. If eating habits can be changed so that a light meal or a salad for dinner is all that is eaten, good, deep rest is a greater possibility. Avoiding rich, sugar-filled desserts can help the sleep process considerably. Complex carbohydrates rather than protein or sweets have proven helpful in inducing sleep. But as simple as these changes are, many alcoholics refuse to budge out of old patterns of behavior. Sleep must be viewed as a precious commodity, and the alcoholic must be willing to do whatever it takes to attain it. If not, sobriety is threatened as the tired and fragile alcoholic finds great difficulty in coping in an exhausted state.

To achieve rest, a regular evening routine needs to be established. Stimuli must be gradually reduced as the hours get later. Meals should be eaten as early as possible, then there should be some relaxing activity such as reading or working a puzzle. Telling oneself to be calm, relax, and prepare for sleep can help. When it is the appropriate time for sleep, go to bed. Do not lie in bed doing other things like sewing or smoking. Just use it to sleep. Establish the routine and stick to it night after night. Implement psychological and physiological solutions to solve the problem. Be sure to get plenty of exercise during the day and plenty of relaxation in the evening. If making those changes does not work, professional help should be sought as soon as possible. A sleep disorder specialist may be the only person who can eliminate what some believe is the number one cause of relapse.

THREAT NUMBER EIGHT: LONELINESS

I touched on loneliness in discussing the second major threat, unhealthy relationships, but it deserves attention as a threat in its own right. Every negative part of a person is magnified through the lens of loneliness. There is nothing healthy about being lonely; it is self-destructive and saps the individual of energy and life. Loneliness must be replaced with supportive relationships and people who care. Recovery does not occur in a vacuum. Isolation from others prevents maturity and growth in the area of emotions. No matter how the alcoholic winds up in a lonely condition, and no matter how few alternatives are seen to the loneliness, he or she must fight to break out of it.

Times of being alone are very beneficial. Everyone needs private space and time to recharge and reenergize, but loneliness is different from productive aloneness. It is a time of insecurity and doubt. There is no sense of meaning or purpose; there is no reason for living when thwarted and trampled by loneliness. Lonely people are not recovering people. It is vitally important to know that anyone can escape the lonely condition.

No one solves loneliness for anyone else. The lonely person must reach out, make an effort to become attached to new activities, search for human contact. Church, civic groups, clubs, and especially AA can be the start of changing a life of loneliness into a meaningful life full of people. Everyone needs encouragement; an occasional supportive pat on the back can produce a positive effect that lasts for days. People can also benefit from being redirected or confronted by others. In relationships with others, life has a chance to exceed expectations. But in a lonely trench of self-degradation, life has no chance.

There are, of course, many who are surrounded by crowds of

people and remain friendless and lonely. These people are miserable because they are cowards. They are afraid to reveal and share the real person on the inside. I call these people "interpersonal wimps." They are spoiled brats and overgrown babies who refuse to take a risk and be real. As a result, they go through life having missed the most valuable part of it. In their emptiness, they drink once again to fill the void.

Loneliness is a killer. To replace it with involvement with others, a professional may be needed, or those who live near a lonely person may have to intervene. The alcoholic may need help in realizing the severity of the situation. Blinded by a self-constructed facade, the lonely person may be totally unaware that the misery can be changed to meaning with the touch of a hand, reaching out to welcome new people and new relationships into his or her life. That touch can be the first step away from the relapse that is often homegrown in a dark corner of loneliness.

THREAT NUMBER NINE: SELF-PITY

Self-pity is a close relative to loneliness. It is a problem of focus. It can be cured with a refocusing of the alcoholic's thoughts and emotions away from the unimportant, back to the essentials that promote progress and growth rather than depression and isolation.

Self-pity comes from making destructive comparisons to other people. When your focus is on others, you often come up short. There is always someone richer, no matter how wealthy you are; there is always someone more attractive, no matter how beautiful you are; there is always someone with more things and a better life-style with fewer problems. If the alcoholic focuses on such people, self-pity is a natural result.

On the other hand, there is always someone worse off, hungrier, poorer, or even uglier. It just depends on where you place your focus whether you come up on top or at the very bottom. But comparison to others does not help anyone; it must be eliminated from recovery altogether. Recovery must be a growing process of doing the best you can with what you have. Accepting limitations and building on strengths makes for a meaningful sobriety. It provides a life of opportunity where how to help others is the focus, rather than figuring out who has more and who has less.

Anyone can be paralyzed by self-pity. It is simple to accomplish. It happens to lazy people who would rather brood over their deficiencies than build on their surpluses. Only the immature are caught up in self-pity. The growing among us have moved on to conquer new worlds of opportunity. They do not have time to compare with others.

Self-pity does not exist where gratitude flourishes. The person who feels inferior must learn to focus on what is good and available. The alcoholic must change to discover the possible rather than brood over and dwell on the impossible. If the alcoholic does not move out of the self-pity mode, it will produce a disastrous result. Eventually, in a fit of self-pity, the alcoholic will develop the attitude of "I might as well be drunk." No alcoholic should let one minute of self-pity endanger the great opportunities found in sobriety and recovery. The move away from relapse starts with a step toward gratitude. Pity belongs only to those who died without a chance to experience recovery—and yet even they often paved the way for someone else to wake up to the need for recovery. Wherever self-pity is alive, a change of focus can kill it and the danger of relapse also.

THREAT NUMBER TEN: OVER-CONFIDENCE

Some enter the recovery process with an unrealistic view of themselves and the disease of alcoholism. They do not fully appreciate just how cunning and baffling this problem really is. They underestimate alcohol's allure, even after months or years of recovery. They forget that to recover, one must be willing to do whatever it takes. They buy into only half or one-fourth of the program. They become overconfident of their ability to recover. So at the point when everything seems to be going perfectly well, when everything appears to be right in place, it all falls apart.

At some point in almost every alcoholic's recovery, there is a desire to be the exception. He or she wants to be the one who can make it without going to Alcoholics Anonymous, or to be the person who can stay close to all the old drinking companions. It is normal to want to be, or to feel like, a unique individual who must adhere only to part of the recovery package.

Just because it is normal, however, does not mean it is helpful. This form of self-confidence is a trap. If it is not replaced with reality, it is an indication of a deeper problem that needs to be resolved.

The recovering alcoholic who insists on tending bar on New Year's Eve, or thinks that AA is not needed, or believes that he or she is "cured" is most likely suffering from a very poor self-image and probably views alcoholism as a moral problem or a sign of weakness. The overconfident covers up what is lacking inside—and that lack is a setup for relapse. Overconfidence must be cut off the moment it is first expressed. It needs to be confronted and challenged by the alcoholic's family and friends. The person must be confronted with the reality of limitations and a complete support system for recovery. If this is not done, it is only a matter of time until the overconfidence results in total collapse of the recovery system.

Not only do feelings about self need to be adjusted; attitudes about alcoholism must be changed. The overconfident alcoholic must learn that strength comes from recovery and not from the denial of the need for recovery. The alcoholic must stop futile battling to prove strength and renew the process of gaining strength. In addition to weakness concepts, problems with the moral view of alcoholism need to be resolved. The alcoholic must be shown, and accept, that moral superiority would not have prevented alcoholism from developing. Equating alcoholism with moral inferiority or weakness creates the need to live recklessly in an overconfident and unrealistic manner.

The overconfident alcoholic is a dishonest alcoholic. Every overconfident act is an attempt to hide the reality of the problem and the reality of the person who has it. Recovery must involve a program of uncompromising honesty. The overconfident alcoholic is living a temporary lie. It is temporary because the lie is shattered when relapse occurs and drinking begins again. No matter what specific component of recovery is being discussed, when you hear an alcoholic claim, "I don't need it," beware. That overconfidence is threatening the hopes of all of those who so desperately want to see alcoholics recover.

The threats to recovery presented here have been felt and experienced by thousands of alcoholics. They are not imaginary; they are real threats that result in relapse. The encouraging aspect of these threats is that they are all preventable. The alcoholic who accepts them as threatening to sobriety can plan to avoid their consequences. Appropriate planning to prevent these threats from destroying recovery can be the foundation of a comprehensive recovery program, a program that produces the freedom and happiness that the alcoholic deserves.

CHAPTER FOURTEEN

COCAINE AND THE CRACK EPIDEMIC

The air was crisp as approaching fall cooled the summer nights of Mundelein, Illinois. A small town outside of Chicago, it is a nice place to raise a family. The schools are excellent and the quality of life high. Families have lots of options for fun and relaxation. But for one family, this was not a night for fun or relaxation. This was a night when reality dashed the dreams of the Bartlett family. The Bartletts suddenly became victims of the epidemic that is striking families across the United States. The epidemic is called crack.

As the sun set and the streetlights flickered on, twelve-year-old Bradley Bartlett biked toward town. His parents had become accustomed to his evening rides. At first they were reluctant to let him ride off alone at dusk, but now they gave it little thought. He always returned by nine o'clock. They imagined that he was merely going to the shopping center, where acres of concrete and asphalt invited skateboarders and bike riders to perfect their stunts. But that was not his destination tonight.

Bradley wanted the thrills that a skateboard or a bike could not offer. Bradley wanted to feel the sensation of crack. He had looked forward to this evening for weeks.

During the weeks just past, Bradley had saved his money. He had managed to gather together fifty dollars for his chemical excursion. Perhaps he had seen kids in movies snort cocaine and smoke crack. Perhaps his friend down the street told him of his own experience, and he formed his plans to experience it also. Maybe he believed it to be fun, exciting, and harmless. Maybe he did not think that being only twelve mattered. He was determined to feel the high that he had heard the media describe.

He knew where to find it, and he had the resources to acquire it. That night he would score.

Bradley pedaled quickly past the crowd of skateboarders at the shopping center, through the downtown traffic lights, and onto a side street that led to a small convenience store. A man was talking in a phone booth outside the store, or at least pretending to talk, to someone on the other end. Bradley circled his bicycle once in front of the store and then stopped on the curb. The man hung up the receiver and walked over to him. The manager of the store watched and would later tell investigators how he had seen something exchange hands between Bradley and the man. A brief discussion ensued, and then Bradley pedaled away.

Two hours later, twelve-year-old Bradley Bartlett was found in the bottom of a dry concrete drainage ditch. Two teenagers going down in the ditch to smoke a joint had found him there. He was motionless and unrevivable. Paramedics could do nothing but transport him to the county morgue. The autopsy revealed the cause of death as drug overdose. Bradley's heart had failed him in his quest for euphoria. Two empty vials, two vials full of crack, a glass pipe and lighter, all found next to Bradley, had indicated the cause of death even before the coroner's knife cut into Bradley's body. The coroner only confirmed the evidence. The purity of the cocaine was too high, producing a physiological effect too intense to survive.

The man in the phone booth was apprehended early the following morning. He had three thousand dollars in his pocket and over a hundred vials of crack in the trunk of his car. A court would prove later that fifty dollars of that three thousand had come from Bradley Bartlett—and that evidence would put Jed Franklin in jail for five years. Being a former high school football letterman couldn't save him from prison. And nothing could save the Bartletts from the horror and grief of losing a son.

Whether by death or addiction, parents are losing their children to the crack epidemic that has swept over this country. Only the naïve believe it is a problem confined to a few larger cities. It is everywhere, and because of its prevalence, this chapter is devoted to this deadly phenomenon. No book on addiction in the eighties would be complete without addressing this national plague that is hurting schools, families, business, and entire communities. Here are some of the basics we need to know to understand and act against the crack epidemic.

STATISTICS

Statistics, even if dry on the surface, are vital to understanding both the magnitude and growth of the cocaine epidemic—and they only verify what those close to the problem already know: the problem is growing and becoming more lethal.

Arnold M. Washton, Ph.D., writing in the *U.S. Journal* in October 1986, stated that over twenty-five million Americans have tried cocaine.[1] Lured by the false image of a harmless, nonaddictive drug, adults, adolescents, and children have been caught up in America's fastest-growing drug problem, and they are learning that just like all the other illicit drugs from the past, the risks are much greater than the pleasures.

The February 1985 issue of *Alcoholism and Addiction Magazine* reported that thirty million people in the United States have tried cocaine and that up to four million are hooked on the drug.[2] *Newsweek*, which has done several excellent cover stories on drugs, cocaine, and crack, made its attempt at quantifying the problem in the Aug. 11, 1986 issue. By using data from the President's Commission on Organized Crime, the National Institute on Drug Abuse, and the Institute for Social Research, it presented the following statistics for 1985:[3]

Twenty to twenty-four million have tried cocaine.
Five million use it regularly.
Five hundred sixty-three have died from it.
Thirty percent try it in college by their fourth year.

Whether twenty million or thirty million have tried it, whether four or five million are hooked, these are staggering numbers, especially compared to a mere half million hard-core heroin users. Some people tend to believe that heroin is the worst of our drug woes, but it is not. It has been overwhelmed by cocaine.

Finally, America appears to be waking up to the severity of the cocaine threat. When the Gallup Organization asked adults which drug presented the most serious problem for society today, 43 percent responded that cocaine and crack combined were the most serious. Thirty-four percent chose alcohol abuse; 5 percent chose heroin, 4 percent marijuana, and 5 percent other drugs. Nine percent didn't know.[4]

Those numbers translate into a mounting problem, one that appears completely out of control. Perhaps the first step toward correcting the problem has been taken: people have finally become aware that it *is* a real problem. Now they must realize that something can and must be done about it. Everyone needs to become involved if we are to turn America's addiction around.

AMERICA'S PROBLEM

Like alcohol addiction, the drug problem cuts across all socioeconomic levels. Nothing has contributed more to its spread than cocaine—first heralded as the glamour drug of the eighties, purported to be a cornucopia of chemical pleasure leaving no addicts in its wake, supposedly a safe drug for all who could afford it. The key to its allure was its high price, which put it out of reach of most Americans—and enhanced its mythology. It was seen as a drug so perfect, so tidy, that the wealthy could use it as if it were a condiment to spice life's pleasures and erase the mundane.

The myth was not easily relinquished. When Richard Pryor cooked up some cocaine to freebase and instead cooked himself, almost burning to death, people continued to believe in the myth and hold to a belief that for all others, it was harmless. When John Belushi mixed heroin and cocaine into a speedball that sped him to his death, the myth survived; Belushi did not. His life-style and carelessness were viewed as the killer, not cocaine.

On June 19, 1986, the rising basketball star Len Bias overdosed on cocaine. His heart, just like Bradley Bartlett's, could not withstand the purity of cocaine. And what was the reaction to his death? Half the kids surveyed by the *New York Times* wrote it off as stupidity, not the danger of the drug.[5] Rather than that he shouldn't have used cocaine, the reaction was that he shouldn't have used it the way he did. So a bright, strong athlete died, but the myth lives on. We have to convince, show, demonstrate, illustrate, teach, and persuade our kids and our fellow adults that cocaine, not the user, is the source of the danger. The evidence is too great, too real to allow anyone to go on believing that no harm comes from this American hobby.

Others have fallen victim to cocaine's seduction. They, unlike the thousands of ghetto-stranded teens strung out on crack, have made the headlines because they are celebrity kids: John Zaccaro, son of the first female vice presidential candidate, arrested for allegedly selling cocaine; Peter Sellers' daughter, Victoria; MacKenzie Phillips; David Kennedy—all names of those who have found out the same things the hard way. Drugs will not take you where you want to go. Cocaine is not a free trip to a joyful paradise. There is a price—there are several prices. Addiction. Jail. Self-worth. Relationships. Businesses. Neighborhoods. Life.

America's problem is not an easy one to solve. Not all the helicopters and soldiers in the American infantry will stamp out our problem in the fields of Bolivia. America must fight the battle with teachers, parents, law enforcement, and legislators on her own soil. America must destroy the mythology of cocaine and replace it with the reality of its dangers. That is how we must begin to eradicate the desire for a high that could kill this country by destroying the potential of the next generation.

PERSPECTIVE

Cocaine is not the first drug to invade this country. No drug other than alcohol has had as many partakers, but other drugs have hurt us and gone on into a decline of popularity, only to be replaced by a more potent or popular chemical. The Civil War brought on an era of morphine addiction; soldiers became addicted when it was used to ease the pain of wounds and amputations. Through much of the nineteenth century, people swigged "tonics" and potent medicines laced with opium (not listed as an ingredient on the labels), which rarely cured illnesses but probably made them (or anything) seem less serious.

World War II seemed to breed a new type of dependency: uppers were taken like candy; amphetamines were used as a daily aid to greater accomplishments and better moods—very like what cocaine users hope to achieve. Their use died down but revived in the sixties. In the meantime, the tranquilizer flooded the medicine chests of America. The fifties introduced thousands to Miltown, and Valium became the most widely prescribed drug ever until Tagamet, an ulcer medication, took the honor.

The psychedelic sixties established drugs as chic, even respectable, with pot as much a middle-class amenity as Scotch. Being stoned was widely regarded as a secular state of grace, and a few generations at once were being sold—and to some extent buying—the gospel of "Tune in, turn on, drop out."

In the seventies, the Vietnam War brought us disappointment, heroin addiction, and more reliance on marijuana. When the eighties rolled in, cocaine became the drug of a new generation. For the eighties, "Coke is It." But it is different from the earlier drugs, because it may not subside. Its popularity, affordability, and availability may not allow for its control unless new tactics and resources are used to fight it.

"We have lost the cocaine battle," Los Angeles police detective Frank Goldberg says.[6] He should know. He is on the front line of the battle. He is a juvenile-narcotics officer in South Central L.A.'s black ghetto.

"The size of the cocaine market is beyond description. It's everywhere." Those are the words of Lieutenant Kunkel. He's not from Los Angeles. He is on the force in Houston, Texas. He says if you stand on any street corner in his town, three people will be there ready to sell you cocaine. All you have to do is ask for it.[7]

Cocaine is making history. Its powers are so pervasive that it could overpower this country. No drug has reached the saturation level and intensity of cocaine. To fight it, we must understand it. To help save our future, we must study this drug's past. We must know it if we are to know its users and how to help them. Few alcoholics would respond to help from someone who did not know what the word "beer" meant. We, in an attempt to help the cocaine victim, must know its meaning also.

Cocaine has been called the champagne of drugs. It is also known as first aid for the rich and famous. It is powerful beyond reason. In one laboratory test, monkeys preferred to take cocaine rather than to live. That should not surprise anyone. Millions are choosing it over life every day. They cannot imagine a life worth living without it.

MORE NUMBERS

The most recent phenomena of cocaine history are the increase in purity and the decrease in price. Comparing the potency of cocaine today to that sold on the street a few years ago is like comparing a roller skate to a locomotive. The cocaine crisis has been magnified by old user habits combined with the purer and more potent cocaine. The combination has proven deadly to many.

Emergency rooms across the country are excellent sources of information about drug-related health emergencies. In those emergency rooms, the number of cocaine-induced illnesses has increased greatly. In 1981, 3,296 were rushed to the local emergency room with cocaine-related problems. That tripled in 1985 to 9,946. In a 1988 study of emergency room admissions related to cocaine, the following results point to the seriousness of cocaine use. Of thirty-nine patients admitted to an E.R., thirteen had acute kidney failure, six died, and eleven had liver malfunction.* This is further proof that cocaine is not an innocent recreational chemical to be considered lightly. The Drug Abuse Warning Network, monitoring twenty-six metropolitan areas, also reported a marked increase in cocaine-related deaths. In 1981, 195 deaths were reported. In the first six months of 1986, the number was already 563.[3] Users simply are not aware of the dangers of the newer high-potency cocaine on the streets today.

Along with the higher purity goes the lower price. A gram of highly cut and less powerful cocaine formerly sold for about a hundred dollars. Now the pure, strong cocaine is selling for less than sixty dollars. Those without sixty dollars can purchase crack for under ten. And those without ten dollars can purchase a dangerous form of cocaine called *bausco* for as little as one dollar a pop. Bausco is a brown paste made from unprocessed coca, the substance that is refined into cocaine. Two years ago, cocaine in any form was not available to buyers in units priced as low as one to ten dollars. The drug of the rich and famous has become available to the poor and unknown, and in a purer form. These two developments—lower price and higher purity— are what have created the cocaine crisis in the last half of the 1980s.

*"In Brief," *Los Angeles Times* (19 September 1988), part 2, 7.

A LOOK BACK

Though the alkaloid cocaine was chemically isolated only in 1860, its source, the coca plant, has been an important, and revered, stimulant and narcotic for thousands of years. In the days of Peru's Inca empire, the coca leaf was chewed to promote endurance, and also as a part of religious ceremonies. It is still so used, though the coca plantations of Peru, Colombia, and Bolivia now produce mainly for the illegal refining and export trade. Cocaine's first use was as a local anesthetic, but its mood-altering effects soon became apparent, and a landmark 1884 paper by Sigmund Freud popularized it as a cure for, of all things, morphine addiction. (An earlier report had told of such a "cure" in the case of a woman who was now perfectly happy to do two weeks on opium and then two weeks on cocaine, and no wonder.) Then as now, cocaine had considerable glamour, and Conan Doyle had Sherlock Holmes at least once inject a 7 percent solution of it to relieve fatigue.

Cocaine was a legal substance in the United States until 1914, when the Pure Food and Drug Act, the Opium Exclusion Act, and the Harrison Narcotic Act wiped out the over-the-counter trade of cocaine and opiates. Before that, the chemical, like opium, was available in cough syrup, elixirs, drinks, and special wines; Abraham Lincoln even bought some. The amount of cocaine was extremely small in the over-the-counter solutions, but even this low level presented problems that finally could be controlled only through regulation.

GETTING THE COCAINE INTO THE BODY

Cocaine can be introduced into the body by snorting, injecting, or smoking it. When cocaine is smoked (inhaled), it enters the system through the tiny capillaries in the lungs. A very intense high results in less than ten seconds that lasts for about fifteen minutes. Smoking cocaine used to require freebasing by heating the cocaine with ignited ether. This dangerous method, the cause of Richard Pryor's burns, hurts the lungs due to the intense heat of the smoke produced. Now inhalation is accomplished by using little rocks that have been broken off from cakes prepared with baking soda and cocaine.

Cocaine is introduced into the system through the mucous

membranes of the nose when it is snorted. This less intense method produces a less intense high that lasts for more than an hour. The other method, injection, is the least effective; much of the cocaine is lost to chemical interaction within the stomach.

Smoking crack or rock cocaine is the method which has been used by the masses to experience the intense, low-cost high— and which has so drastically intensified the cocaine crisis.

THE CRACK CRISIS

Cocaine in the form of crack is more deadly and crippling than anyone ever imagined. Crack is *different*. Robert M. Stutman, special agent in charge of the Drug Enforcement Administration of the New York region, declares, "What makes crack different from all other drugs is the unbelievably quick potential for addiction."[9] According to Arnold Washton, "If a sinister master chemist or a sinister pharmacologist wanted to invent a drug that would addict large numbers of people at low cost, I don't think he could do any better than this one."[10]

The onset of crack addiction occurs so early in the use of crack because of the intense high from the drug and the crashing low that produces deep depression when the drug's effect wears down. In the midst of that deep depression, the cocaine addict reaches out to soar again. The run from depression leads back to repeated use; the repeat only produces greater postcocaine dysphoria and locks the user deeper into addiction. A cycle develops in which craving and hunger for the chemical engulf the user's willpower. Within less than two weeks a user can become an addict. That quick rush to addiction is not paralleled by any other drug.

Our society is being ravaged by the effects and side effects of cocaine. This drug is so powerful that a son will forge his parents' name onto a grant deed and sell their house for money to buy cocaine. A mother will use it as an aid to lose weight and find it socially acceptable to discuss it with friends. A hardworking carpenter will abandon his craft and his family, lured into cocaine dealing by the hopes of making a bundle of money.

Clinical psychologist Ruth Stafford, a specialist in treating cocaine addiction and chemical dependency, says that it is in all the high schools. It is no longer an elitist drug associated with the high rollers. Truck drivers and roofers as well as mothers and their school-age children are being swept into the addiction cycle.[11]

In the summer of 1986 it began to seem, in cities across the country, that the war against crack was being lost. In New York it was called the long, hot summer of crack. The highly purified cocaine became so prevalent that law enforcement officials claimed to be powerless to stop it. The courts were jammed, and treatment centers were filled to capacity. Teenage dealers sold to ten-year-olds as the epidemic mushroomed into a nightmare.

New York District Attorney Robert M. Morgenthau, Jr., stated, "Once I thought we were treading water; now I feel we are drowning."[12] Not a person or neighborhood is immune. The dealers are in suburban parks and in downtown business districts, and crack houses that distribute the chunks of purified cocaine and baking soda can be found anywhere. They have become as commonplace as a chain of stereo stores. They are mom-and-pop operations that have become a lucrative cottage industry for thousands of dealers. Teenagers are becoming wealthy from dealing. Too young to drive, they have chauffeured BMWs, because they are not too young to deal. Abundant, quick money has brought crack into every level of society.

The damage to society also comes in the form of crime. In many communities where crime was on the decline, it is now increasing rapidly. Crack and crack dealing are the major causes of the increase. Wherever crack is, there is vicious violence between the dealers and users, along with an increase in petty crime. In New York, police believe that crack is the primary cause of the 18 percent increase in robbery.[13]

When a community is hit by crack, it becomes involved in a guerrilla war that police find almost impossible to control. Pushers, dealers, couriers, and lookouts work together to form a distribution network employing kids and teenagers. When the police attack these well-organized systems of illegal commerce, the network can quickly disappear. Crack is flushed down toilets, and not enough evidence is left for prosecution. Because the courts and prisons are so full, punishment is rare. If the war on crack is to be won, sure punishment must become the rule, but even when crack dealers are punished, they often return to the street quickly to continue their trade.

Neighborhoods are being overrun by the crack trade, but residents are apathetic. They expect the police to do something but are unwilling to police themselves. The residents are afraid to act. They fear retaliation from dealers if they prosecute or testify against them, so the justice system and law enforcement have been impotent to thwart the menace to our children.

As a result of law enforcement's inability to control the problem, the crack business has little risk. It also has high monetary rewards. Organized crime has not yet taken over this branch of the drug industry. The small dealer can get in relatively cheaply and make a quick profit. An ounce of cocaine purchased for six hundred dollars can be turned into 168 rocks that will sell for over two thousand dollars. The dealer doubles the investment in a very short time.

Kids who just sit in a crack house for seven hours can earn three hundred dollars in one day. That much money at the risk of being busted is seen as a fair bet. Los Angeles Police Department Detective Steve Havel says that the kids are able to live out the *Miami Vice* fantasy; they wear heavy gold jewelry and sweatshirts costing two hundred dollars or more, drive a Mercedes or Lamborghini, and see the world through hundred-and-sixty dollar Porsche sunglasses. And where there is money, there is violence. So many rubouts and rip-offs have happened in Oakland, California, that it has been called "Beirut without tanks." In three years there have been fifty-seven drug-related deaths.[14] More neighborhoods are going to be hit by the crack plague if new strategies are not devised to stop the crime and corruption produced by the little white rocks. But the toll cannot be reckoned by a survey of neighborhoods. It is only accurately assessed when individuals who use it are studied. The high is personal, and the hurt is personal also.

COCAINE'S PERSONAL EFFECTS

Emotional Effects

The single reason for cocaine's widespread popularity is the way the drug makes people feel. With crack, those feelings are heightened to the extreme. Cocaine stimulates the central nervous system. Taken in small doses, it produces an energetic feeling; the tired become awake and alert. For the moment, the effect appears to be superior to that of a chemical-free existence. But the following day brings lethargy and depression. Rarely acknowledged by users, those, too, are part of the package of feelings produced by cocaine. They cause the peak performer to sag into ineffectiveness the day after.

Crack really does heighten the highs and deepen the lows. It stretches the emotional boundaries like no other chemical. As one addict said about the intense rush, "It goes straight to the head. It's immediate speed; it feels like the top of your head is going to blow off."[15] Crack is absorbed very quickly through the capillaries in the lungs and goes through the blood to the brain within seconds. This quick rise to euphoria causes the crash to depression. It also intensifies the paranoia and suspiciousness that accompany repeated use of cocaine. The anxiety, concentration difficulties, depression, and paranoia far outweigh the early pleasure of cocaine use. The price for the cocaine high is an emotional roller coaster ride that many do not survive.

Physical Effects

The entire physiology of the body is altered by the use of cocaine. Crack racks the body even harder and hurts it quicker. The user of crack has chronic sore throats and is constantly hoarse. Short of breath, often gasping for air, the cocaine user manifests lung damage. Long-term use leads to emphysema, and respiratory arrest can be caused by an overdose.

The cardiovascular system is even more severely affected. Blood pressure and heart rate increases lead to arrhythmia—irregular heartbeat—or even a heart attack. The stimulation also adversely affects the brain. Paranoia psychosis similar to schizophrenia results from long-term use; a short-term danger from brain overstimulation is seizure and convulsions. Users also lose their appetite. The desire for food is depressed, and weight loss, even malnutrition, results.[16]

Cocaine does nothing wonderful for the body. It puts it under stress that causes early aging; dry skin is only one manifestation of a body undernourished and overtaxed. Life in the cocaine fast lane draws life out of its user.

Observable Symptoms

What can you observe when someone is using cocaine? How do you decide that the personal changes and deterioration are a result of cocaine? The following is a list of symptoms that the cocaine user may exhibit. Of course, many may be symptoms of other problems, but cumulatively, they spell out drug dependency from cocaine and crack use.[17]

- Sniffling, runny nose, nosebleeds, sinus infections, preoccupation with and touching of the nose
- Hoarseness, coughing, respiratory infections, throat clearing, respiratory problems
- Loss of weight
- Dark circles under the eyes
- Pale skin
- Tremor and nervous twitches
- Pupil dilation
- Talking about being depressed
- Talking about financial problems
- Loss of interest in important things
- Apathy
- Paranoia
- Repeating conversations
- Incomplete ideas and rapid changes of topic
- Rapid, choppy speech
- Forgetfulness
- Absenteeism
- Tardiness
- Temper tantrums
- Insomnia and fatigue
- Speedy, compulsive behavior
- Extreme mood swings
- Reduction of outside interests
- Isolation from friends
- Decrease in appetite

Progressive Symptoms

Cocaine has a progression that leads directly to addiction. It starts with experimental use, moves to social use, and then to habitual use. From there it is on to addiction. But with crack, it is not uncommon for addiction to start with the first use.

The reason for the quick move into addiction is the rapid development of high tolerance. The high tolerance leads the user into uncontrollable use before the user knows that control has been lost. The individual is rushed to a state where controlled use is impossible. Any wish for abstinence is disrupted by craving and cocaine hunger, and the addiction completely dominates the addict's life.

Addiction is identified by four major signs. One is the compulsion to use again and again. The second is the loss of control; the compulsive use cannot be stopped as long as the supply is near. The third sign of addiction is the continued use even though adverse consequences become more and more obvious. As with other addictions, denial is a significant characteristic.

Arnold Washton outlines the clinical characteristics of cocaine dependence as follows:[18]

Loss of controlled use
- Inability to refuse the drug when offered
- Inability to assess the amount of use
- "Binge" patterns of excessive use for twenty-four hours or longer
- Unsuccessful attempts to stop usage for a significant length of time

Drug compulsion
- Persistent or episodic cravings and compulsions
- Compulsive use despite absence of drug-induced euphoria
- Compulsions stronger than desire to stop usage
- Fears of being without cocaine
- Compulsion to use other drugs in absence of cocaine

Continued use despite adverse consequences
- Medical complications: lethargy, insomnia, nasal or sinus problems, appetite disturbance, loss of sex drive, impotence
- Psychiatric complications: depression, irritability, anhedonia, paranoia, suicidal/homicidal tendencies
- Social and financial complications, legal or job problems, general deterioration in psychosocial functioning

Denial
- Denial that the problem exists
- Denial or downplaying of the seriousness of adverse effects
- Defensive actions in response to inquiries about drug use

The progression toward the bottom is predictable. The following are some milestones along the way. Not everyone experiences these problems in just this exact order or intensity, but these markers are common to many involved in the cocaine addiction battle.

Initial Stage
- Introduction to cocaine in some form
- Only uses when offered
- Stimulation in social settings
- Discovery of the effects of the drugs

Regular Usage
- Starts to purchase on own
- Used to heighten sexual experiences
- All-night binges
- Financial regrets after all-nighters
- Buying cocaine to stockpile it

Dependent Usage
- Work performance hurt
- Dealing to supply self
- Loss of outside interests
- Willpower destroyed
- Change in companions
- Unable to stop while supply lasts
- Paranoid episodes
- Grandiose behavior
- Solitary use of cocaine

Addictive Usage
- Missing parties because of cocaine's unavailability
- Unkept promises to quit
- Lack of sexual abilities
- Unending search for more cocaine
- Work and financial problems
- Overdose
- Physical deterioration

Late Stage
- Frequent long binges
- Inability to quit
- Isolation from family and friends
- Paranoia and hallucinations
- Impaired thinking

- Moral degradation
- Financial collapse
- Loss of family
- Bizarre behavior

All addictive chemicals progress into a severe stage of uncontrolled use and complete deterioration of life-style, but crack's edge on the rest is its ability to hook and addict quickly. This makes its progression much more dangerous and deadly; millions have become trapped before they knew how dangerous the drug was.

ADDITIONAL DANGERS

As if the preceding problems were not enough, there are other disasters created by crack and cocaine. One of the worst is the increase in the number of babies born hooked on cocaine. The number of babies born with cocaine in the bloodstream has jumped ten times in one year, as reported in some hospitals. The babies are born in emotional turmoil, their emotions on edge. They have to be sedated with Valium, phenobarbital, or even Thorazine. Other cocaine babies just lie motionless, unable to breathe unassisted.[19]

A study done in 1988, the first detailed study of babies that had been exposed to cocaine before birth, revealed the severe damage done to the fetus by cocaine. The study revealed an epidemic of damaged infants, some impaired for life from a brief use of cocaine during pregnancy. The cocaine babies exhibited:

- retarded growth in the womb
- subtle neurological abnormalities
- loss of small intestine
- brain damaging strokes
- a tendency to die or be born prematurely
- smaller bodies, heads and brains
- genital deformities*

*"Cocaine: Litany of Fetal Risks Grows," *New York Times* (6 September 1988) 19.

Pregnant women must be taught, motivated, and even begged to stay away from this drug.

Another danger is death of the babies of mothers who use cocaine and crack. At one hospital, there were two in one day. One mother of a cocaine baby said, "I made a big mistake, and I want people to know that you shouldn't do this to your child. You've just got to get yourself together and get help, or you and your child are going to suffer."[20]

Add to all of these problems the car accidents and suicides brought about by cocaine use, and the immense dangers become obvious. The epidemic is severe and its consequences are terrible, but there is hope. The hope lies in treatment of the addict. When treatment is obtained, recovery is possible.

TREATMENT AND RECOVERY

No one should expect addicted people to be able to pull themselves out of an addiction problem and into recovery. Cocaine addiction, with its intense high and slick mythology, is even harder to abandon. It is common for kids to be admitted to treatment kicking and screaming, yet to end up finding hope through recovery. What a person says in the throes of addiction is not a true indication of the desires underneath.

Three important elements of treatment are essential for recovery. First, the person must get the cocaine out of the system. The body must be allowed to return to normal. The second element involves a positive support system. This support system should start with a treatment team and expand to family and friends. This support system must educate, provide therapy, and reinforce the recovery process. The third aspect of treatment involves the establishment of rewarding things to do, things that provide meaning and satisfaction. If the person is not going to get high, something must fill the void. All three elements of treatment are very important in establishing a strong recovery program.

Recovery is never over for the addict. It is a process that involves continual follow-up to prevent relapse. An essential of the follow-up is involvement with a group such as Cocaine Anonymous, Narcotics Anonymous, or Alcoholics Anonymous. The long-term recovery process is the same as that presented earlier in this book. It is not different from that for an alcoholic. There are other similarities between the person addicted to alcohol and the person addicted to cocaine.

COCAINE AND ALCOHOL ADDICTION CORRELATIONS

In the eighties, the major similarity between alcohol and cocaine is that they are both very social drugs. They are often used with each other in the same settings. They serve as a buffer from each other, one acting as a stimulant, the other as a sedative. In addition, few use cocaine who have not used alcohol. Alcohol, tobacco, and marijuana are the gateway drugs to heroin and cocaine. Children in particular use alcohol before moving to cocaine.

Whichever comes first, cocaine and alcohol promote each other. When the cocaine crash hits, the user will grab anything to help, and alcohol is used most frequently to ease the crash because of its common accessibility.

Any addiction problem results from a combination of genetics and environment. Different people react differently to different drugs. Few, about 20 percent, appear to have inherited an addictability to alcohol. The percentage who have an addictability to cocaine is unknown, but it is very high. Both drugs develop tolerance in the user, and both drugs have a withdrawal syndrome when use is discontinued. They both result in uncontrolled use. And when controlled use is attempted for either addict, relapse results.

The biggest similarity between the two is that both react chemically with the brain to produce pleasure. And as long as people experience that pleasure, they will abuse the chemicals. Some with systemic propensities go on to become addicted. Few who use alcohol become addicted; most who use cocaine regularly do.

No other industrialized country has an addictive problem as severe as ours. Right now the fastest-growing contributor to that problem is cocaine in the form of crack. It is time that something is done to curb the rise in addiction and the problems that result from it. It is time for everyone to admit a problem exists. Affluent schools must abandon their drive to achieve recognition as model schools and admit the prevalence of the drug dilemma.

The schools' refusal to admit the existence of the problem is a major barrier to dealing with it, but parents' denial is an even greater one. It is difficult to motivate parents to recognize the symptoms of drug use and addiction; each parent must finally be willing to admit that "it can happen to my child."

No longer can we accept that recreational use is harmless. Recreational use is where the drug epidemic begins. We cannot tolerate it among kids or our fellow adults. We need to make a commitment to solve the problem once and for all. Money, time, and effort must be dedicated to the war. It is not too late. It is a battle that can be won, but more must jump into the fray. It is the only battle that has no combat victims; the victim count only rises when no one is willing to fight.

NOTES

1. Arnold M. Washton, "Teen Use Increasing," *U.S. Journal of Alcohol and Drug Dependency*, vol. 9, no. 10 (October 1985): 9.
2. "Cocaine: The Deadliest Cargo," *Alcoholism and Addiction Magazine* (February 1986): 17.
3. Larry Martz et al., "Try To Say No," *Newsweek* (11 August 1986): 15.
4. Ibid., 16.
5. "New York City Being Swamped by Crack," *Los Angeles Times* (1 August 1986), part 1, 22.
6. "Kids and Cocaine," *Newsweek* (17 March 1986), 60.
7. Ibid.
8. "New York City Being Swamped By Crack," *Los Angeles Times*.
9. Peter Kerr, "New Form of Cocaine Brings Renewed Concern Over Drugs," *Orange County Register* (10 August 1986), A17.
10. *Alcoholism and Addiction Magazine* (February 1986): 19.
11. "County's Affluent Attracts Growing Cocaine Trade." *Los Angeles Times* (26 January 1986), part II, 5.
12. "New York City Being Swamped by Crack," *Los Angeles Times*.
13. "Crack and Crime." *Newsweek* (16 June 1986), 16.
14. Janice Castro, "Buried by a Tropical Snowstorm," *Time* (17 March 1986), 62.
15. Jacob V. Lamar, Jr., "Crack," *Time* (2 June 1986), 16.
16. Ibid.
17. Marc B. Becker, "Cocaine and the Workplace," *The Messenger*, vol. 1, no. 12 (December 1986): 1, 7.

18. Arnold M. Washton, *Cocaine Abuse Treatment Psychiatry Letter*, vol. III, issue 9 (September 1985).

19. "Cocaine Babies: Hooked at Birth." *Newsweek* (28 July 1986), 56.

20. Ibid., 57.

CHAPTER FIFTEEN

AN EPIDEMIC OF ENABLING

America and other countries around the world are experiencing an epidemic of addiction for one reason: there is an epidemic of enabling found in almost every area of our society. No addict can continue to be addicted unless a system allows the addiction to continue. Family, friends, counselors, ministers, teachers, employers, community leaders, law enforcement personnel, and attorneys all play a part in allowing junkies to drug and alcoholics to drink. When everyone works together to stop enabling, addiction can be controlled. For this to happen, new behaviors must be learned. These behaviors are more difficult than enabling behaviors, but they produce change. They make people accountable for what is happening in their lives; they confront every alcoholic and addict with the consequences of their behavior; they no longer hide, cover, or deny the reality of a sick individual or a sick community.

Enabling is any assistance given to an alcoholic or an addict that hides, covers, removes, or minimizes the harmful consequences of alcoholism and drug addiction. The motives of the enabler are not bad; the intention is to help the addict. But good intentions do not end up in resolving addiction. It takes corrective action that may be painful now but produces the desired results later. The "quick fix" does not help, either. Fast cures only produce false hopes that never lead to long-term recovery. No matter how hard the enabler tries to "fix" the addict or the world around the addict, the effort always ends in disappointment. When enabling stops, the disappointment subsides and real hope dawns.

Enabling starts out as denial. There is a complete rejection

of the fact that a problem exists. Schools will deny a problem
so that their administrations will not be viewed as incompetent;
businesses deny it so that shareholders will not become alarmed;
and certain professions deny the problem because of pride. But
the evidence in recent years has erased much of the denial that
caused inaction. From baseball to boardrooms, people are forced
to accept the existence of a problem and to do something about
it. No longer are most organizations able to say "It can't happen
here."

Even though the problem is more widely recognized, enabling continues. Just recognizing the problem does not solve
it. Rationalization and projection are just as deadly as denial.
Blaming someone else for the problem does not help resolve it.
Pointing fingers at law enforcement or school systems does
nothing but delay the needed corrective action.

PARENTS

Enabling begins at home. It must also end there. Parents of
addicted children refuse to believe that their children are capable
of having a problem. So they overlook evenings that end in a
night of vomiting and a "sudden virus." They accept the kids'
irrational lies that are attempts to cover up the problem. As
enablers, parents look at the symptoms of a problem and try to
manage them, rather than attempting to correct the source. Parents also try to blame rather than take action. They look to the
other parent, the school, or the town for the reason for the trouble. The sooner parents make an honest appraisal of their children, the sooner some can be saved from the progression of
addiction.

Parents enable their children because they care about
them. They want to make life easier and more manageable.
They will go to great lengths to try to provide the best for
their kids. Believing that the problems surrounding the child
will pass, they try to make life more comfortable while the
child struggles to mature. It is human nature to do that; if
someone has a cold or a virus, it is natural to take responsibility away from them. To pamper and care for them in a
loving way, until the illness passes, is a proper way to help
someone in that condition. But it does not work well with

a child addict. Home remedies and making life easier do not help but only allow the addiction process to tighten its grip on the child.

Parents must stop enabling and own the responsibility of dealing with addiction. It is not a phase and must be identified as something that one does not magically grow out of. Every parent with a problem youngster, whether six years old or twenty-six, must accept the strong possibility that drugs or alcohol may be the source of the problem. The way to begin to analyze the possibility is to talk rationally to the child, not just once, but many times. Often, after repeated discussions, lies stop and the truth comes out.

Many parents feel incompetent to deal with their adolescent's problems. In that case, they must consult with professionals who have been trained in both adolescent treatment and chemical dependency. A professional can help a parent sort through the lies presented by the young addict. The professional can help the parents to act consistently, not in an enabling way, but in a corrective way. The parents can learn to help the adolescent see the obvious consequences of destructive behavior.

Let us consider the example of an affluent child who has an automobile, money to ski, money to date, and ample freedom. Everything is going well until the parents notice the grades start to drop. The parents must act to motivate better grades. If drugs or drunkenness caused the deteriorating grades, the child is forced to make a choice. Mom and Dad lay out a plan. If the grades go up, the car is still the kid's. If the grades stay the same or plummet, the car will magically disappear. To ensure that they go up, no skiing until the next grades come out. This gives the child a message early in the development of the problem. The message is that if certain things happen, a price must be paid. Consequences must be addressed and realized.

If the parents do not see improvement in both performance and attitude, they should strongly suspect that something more than a behavior problem exists. They should consider the possibility of drug involvement. Ask the question: "What is powerful enough to motivate a child to give up a car, skiing, and freedom?" There are not many things other than booze and drugs. The next step would be to take the child to a counselor experienced in handling drug and alcohol problems. The counselor can sort through the pieces of the problem and develop a plan to assist the family and the adolescent.

The most important thing for parents to remember is that early action is vital. There can come a time when the child is so out of control that nothing can be done. The adolescent ends up in prison for stealing because he or she was caught trying to support a habit. The sooner the parents intervene in the addict's life, the better. The action must not focus only on the young addict; it must include the relationship with the parents as well as with brothers or sisters. Everyone must accept the responsibility of getting involved in the change process and of supporting it.

When this happens, it is amazing what a profound impact can be produced on the world. One adolescent getting help motivates others to seek help also. Save an adolescent from addiction and you stop the cycle from being repeated in his or her own future family. At least you create a greater potential of avoiding that cycle. No matter how painful it is, the parents must look realistically at the evidence of addiction in the lives of every child they are attempting to raise. By facing the pain now, disaster is avoided later. What appears incredibly difficult today makes for a much easier future. No one can act for the parent. Each parent must take action to do something today; tomorrow is often too late.

THE SCHOOL SYSTEM

Another area where enabling abounds is the school system. A perfect example is here in Southern California. One of the high schools was in the running to be one of the top schools in the United States. The administration and teachers wanted this honor; as a result, they refused to admit the problem of drugs on campus. They would not address it openly; they would deny it publicly. Nothing could budge these people into taking responsibility for facing the problem. Their image was too important. That kind of irresponsible attitude is displayed all the time.

Enabling is not just a problem in high schools; it can be found in schools from elementary levels to universities. The most common defense the school system uses is that it is someone else's problem. It believes that the parents should take care of it at home. School officials make statements like "It is the job of the school to teach; it is not the job of the school to cure society of what ails it." When it comes to society's drug problem, it *is* the school's job to help. It must help by implementing a program that allows nonusing kids, free of alcohol and drugs, to go to school without pressure to use, and also motivates those who are not users to accept help for the problem. The school must not take the route of expulsion or punishment as a first line of action. It must have a comprehensive program to help kids stay clean.

Where does a program for the schools begin? With the parents and teachers. Parents must be made aware of the extent of drug use on campus. They must be educated on the signs and symptoms of drug use and alcoholism. They need to be encouraged not to cover up the problem and enable their youngsters. Parents need to understand what the school will be doing to help kids with alcohol and drug problems. Parents and teachers must consider themselves part of a coalition designed to help kids, not hurt them. They must be taught the steps needed to confront the problem.

Simultaneously with an educational program for parents and teachers, the school should implement a program that intervenes early in a student's drug use and provides a way for the young person to receive help. A good program is very simple to form and implement. The program in the school, just like a program in a place of employment, is based on performance. The student whose grades fall, attendance drops, or tardiness increases is referred to a committee to assess the problem. This committee is not established to diagnose alcoholism and drug addiction. It is designed to assess the evidence of a person's record and recommend action. It should be composed of students, teachers, parents, and administrators if it is to be truly effective.

When a name is sent to the committee, a date is set for the student to appear before it. Before that date, a survey on that student is passed on to the parents and teachers, who answer questions about attitude, behavioral problems, and suspected drug use and drinking. The student is also asked to submit a summary of why he or she believes that performance has declined and a plan to correct the problem. When the committee meets with the student, it reviews all such information, along with the student's records. The committee's findings and recommendations are then sent to the parents to gain their agreement to the remedial plan decided on.

The plan might be as simple as required study time after school; it cannot be assumed that drugs are always the cause of a decline in school performance. The student, given extra attention, is allowed to improve. But if performance does not improve, another meeting is scheduled to plan a new course of action. Plans always include a review and follow-up session to track progress. When progress is not forthcoming, a new plan must be implemented. Other plan elements could include attending alcohol and drug education classes. There could also be the inclusion of a visit to a counselor with the parents. When the evidence obviously points toward a drug and alcohol problem, recommendation for treatment might be made.

For a plan to be effective, parents, teachers, and administration must all accept the concept and support it completely, even when it involves one of the parents' own children. This type of comprehensive program must include the following key elements if it is to make a successful effort to stop alcohol and drugs in schools:

Cooperation by parents, teachers, and administration
Education of parents, teachers, students, and administration
Assessment of students whose performance deteriorates
Implementation of a plan to correct the problem
Intervention when alcohol and drugs are apparently part of the problem
Referral to appropriate resources when outside help is needed
Follow-up to assure that appropriate action has been taken
Evaluation of the program by parents, teachers, and students on a continuing basis

The program must not overlook one very important concept that damages many programs that do overlook it. Whatever is illegal should be punished appropriately. Minors who drink often break the law. No committee should prevent appropriate punishment when the law is broken. Drinking while driving is not something for a committee to handle; it is a crime to be dealt with by the legal system. The same holds true for illicit drug use and dealing; that is something for the courts to punish and correct. If the courts have an effective program, the corrective action will include more than punishment. The school program is for those problems that do not come under the banner of illegality.

When a school system enforces a thorough plan to correct the alcohol and drug problem, the entire community benefits, and a lot of misery is avoided. It is easy to transfer children with alcohol or drug problems to other school districts; it is also easy to expel them from school; it is even easier simply to punish the offenders. Easy is not always best. In this case, what is easy is also irresponsible. The responsible way of handling the problem is to implement a plan that motivates kids, teachers, administrators, and parents to take corrective action and initiate change.

THE LEGAL SYSTEM

The entire legal system must become involved in a coordinated effort to stop enabling alcoholism and drug addiction. At every level there must be responsible action to correct the problem rather than allow it to escalate. From police officers to attorneys to judges, everyone must be committed not only to punishing those who break the law but to treating addicts and alcoholics so there is no longer a need to break the law. Repeat offenders not given an opportunity to get well will continue to be repeat offenders. But a good, solid plan can change the lives of many of those people.

Let's look at the case of the prominent businessman who is stopped for driving while intoxicated. If the police officer is a friend of the family, he might not arrest the driver. In what is meant as an effort to help, the officer might just drive the man home. If charges are filed, there will probably be an attorney dedicated to getting them dropped. In many locales a judge will reduce the charges or dismiss the case. All of these are enabling behaviors that allow people to escape the consequences of dangerous actions. Drunk driving kills, and

everyone must be committed to stopping it and getting the
drunk driver off the road—not only off the road but into treatment for the problem.

In a legal system designed to help people with drug and
alcohol problems, no one gets off the hook. The mayor's
daughter has no way out of punishment—and help—if caught
using drugs; the minister's son is not allowed to settle a drug-
pushing charge out of court; there are no plea bargains that
enable problems to increase. Rather than letting anyone off,
everyone entering the system must be offered treatment as a
part of sentencing. By the time a person's problem reaches
the level at which the courts are involved, education is too
late. Classes are not effective. People need treatment for the
problem.

The attorney's role is integral in diverting people from
tragedy or allowing them to sink further into it. The detrimental act of getting drunk drivers off is not the only unhealthy thing that attorneys do; they can enable the problem
in other ways. Take the couple who are divorcing over a
drinking problem. The attorney must be committed to help
the people, not just take money for filling out papers. The
lawyer must ask about alcohol, and when it is involved, must
make the appropriate referral to resolve the problem. Anything less than referral for treatment when alcoholism is evident is irresponsible. Fortunately, many attorneys refuse to
neglect the need to help people. They take the responsibility
of finding appropriate help for their clients, at least recom-
mending it.

Each element of the legal system needs a referral-and-
treatment component. True justice, combined with the opportunity to change, is the best example a community's legal
system can set for kids. Everyone must know that if the law
is broken, punishment is the result, and the community leaders must ensure that, in addition to punishment, treatment
alternatives are available for those who need them.

COMMUNITY LEADERS

Community leaders can lead the entire community away from
enabling toward handling the drug and alcohol problem that

exists in each locality. They must ensure that the community can offer the elements needed to combat the problem. They must also ensure that people in need are motivated to take advantage of those elements. Communities with successful drug and alcohol programs utilize the following components:

PUBLIC AWARENESS: Public awareness can be increased through the media. A coordinated campaign to raise awareness of alcoholism, drunk driving, and drug addiction involves radio, television, and newspapers.

EDUCATION: Education programs for the public are funded. These programs of lectures and educational experiences can be handled by schools, hospitals, clinics, health clubs, and community groups. A good campaign strives to get every citizen to attend at least one program.

PREVENTION: Prevention goes beyond education. Prevention programs involve a commitment from each sector of the community. Bars and restaurants must know to take appropriate action when drunkenness occurs. Businesses, schools, legal system, and community groups must all be committed to preventing addiction and other alcohol- and drug-related problems.

TREATMENT: Community leaders need to support private treatment centers. Each one that exists means that fewer tax dollars are needed to fund other treatment resources, needed for those who do not have money or insurance to cover the cost of private treatment. Publicly funded treatment centers should stand alongside the private ones to help alcoholics and addicts recover. Halfway houses should be built and run so that people in need of longer-term support can have it. If treatment is not available, nothing will effectively help a community with its problem. It is the most important element in a comprehensive program. No community is too small; according to conservative figures, about 20 percent of the population has an alcohol or drug problem. In a town of a thousand, that is at least two hundred people in need of help, help the community leaders can make sure is available.

THE EMPLOYERS

By now, most major employers have a formalized employee assistance program for alcohol and drug problems. They offer help when people's job performance deteriorates through alcohol or drug abuse. But major employers are not the only ones who need a program; every business needs a program of some sort to help employees with their problems. It is not only a very humane thing to do, it saves the business money by reducing sick time and increasing productivity. Without a program, a company loses money and a lot of potentially good employees.

Enabling in business occurs in many different forms. One of the most common is a supervisor covering up the problem by doing the work for the employee. There are many motives for doing this. It allows the supervisor to feel like a "savior" to the subordinate. The supervisor may also do it out of guilt: the alcoholic or addict may be able to successfully convince the supervisor that the work is too hard or that the supervisor has driven too much. Falling into this trap, the supervisor may feel the need to take up the slack for the problem worker, but doing that only prolongs everyone's agony.

Another very damaging form of enabling occurs constantly at higher levels of organizations. An executive with the company a long time who develops a drinking problem is often treated differently from other employees. The damage is inflicted on that person when expectations are lowered and the person is essentially warehoused until death or retirement. Ask the president if there is a drinking problem in the company, and he or she will point to this person. Everyone is aware of the problem. Think of the needless damage to this person's self-esteem, family, and future by the pervasive expectation that there will be no change. This form of enabling should be eliminated from every business.

The nonenabling plan for business is very simple. It involves the elements of education, documentation, intervention, and referral. First, the employees need to be educated about what is normal drinking, what is alcohol abuse, and what is alcoholism. The plan must also educate the employees about the availability of help when trouble is encountered.

That help should be readily available to employees and the families.

The second element is documentation of performance. When that performance drops, the employee should be counseled and given a plan to improve. When performance does not improve, intervention should take place, and the employee should be referred to an appropriate resource. If the problem involves alcohol or drugs, the appropriate resource is treatment.

Attitudes at work are important for long-term recovery. Everyone needs to be on the side of the recovering addict. The employer should sponsor recovery groups so that every employee knows that management is supportive of recovery and of those who need help.

In concluding this section on employers, it is important to comment on drug screens and drug tests. Any company or organization that is willing to go to the expense should be entitled to this procedure. There are some jobs and professions where it should be a requirement: flying passenger aircraft, medicine, and other occupations in which people's lives are at stake. Professional sports is another area where testing is completely appropriate. It allows management to keep organized crime from controlling the game and players through the use of drugs. It also ensures that these influential professionals will set a positive example for the thousands of kids who admire them. Drug tests or not, every organization needs a plan to help with alcohol and drug problems. When business stops enabling at every level, society takes a giant step toward solving its alcohol and drug problem.

PHYSICIANS

Physicians are trained to help people ease the pain of illness and disease; sometimes, rather than help an addict or an alcoholic, the physician enables him. Enabling can come in the form of prescribing sleeping pills over a long period of time. If the sleep disorder is not corrected in a short time, the pills will not help; they will only lead the person into addiction. Tranquilizers are also a trap often initiated by the physician. A quick prescription can result in a lifetime of addiction. Indiscriminate prescribing of mood-altering drugs must be replaced with careful consideration and concern; this certainly also applies to the prescription of diet pills.

When alcoholism is a possibility, the doctor must be willing to ask about drinking. When tests and symptoms point toward heavy drinking, the physician must risk confrontation. That risk is a financial one since the person may decide to change doctors, but the responsible physician is more concerned with health and living than preservation of a patient base.

If the symptoms become apparent, the physician should act to help the person. That help might take the form of a consultation with a psychologist; it could also mean a gathering of the family to confront the patient with the need for treatment. To help with alcohol and drug problems, a minimal level of assistance is at least to ask about and assess that area of a person's life. When the evidence is strong for alcohol or drug abuse, the physician can be a powerful force for change and treatment. Often people who will not take advice from anyone will listen to a doctor. The credibility of the physician is hard to match.

THE MINISTER

A study of alcoholics in treatment revealed that the clergy, more than any other professionals were approached for help somewhere during the progression of alcoholism. Ministers came in contact with more alcoholics and drug abusers than any other identified source of help. Yet few referrals to treatment come from ministers. The reason is the philosophical base from which many in the clergy operate. Not understanding the true nature of alcoholism, the minister will often prescribe prayer and other methods for spiritual growth. Some will attempt healing of the alcoholic. Often the results are instant but not permanent. They do not last because only the spiritual dimension is addressed, and recovery must be multidimensional.

Another reason that ministers do not refer alcoholics into treatment is the fear of driving a parishioner out of the church. They are afraid that AA or some other organization will replace the role of the church in the person's life. This is a possibility if the minister is not involved in the process of recovery. But when he is involved, the alcoholic will not replace church with anything. The alcoholic or addict will see church as a key component of spiritual recovery.

Some ministers continue to deny the existence of alcohol and drug problems in their congregation. But any church with teenagers has a drug and alcohol problem. Every day these kids are up against an incredible pressure to drink and use. Some of them, even those who attend church every week, succumb to the pressure. Another source of the problem is evident in women or men who attend church alone. Many do so because there is a drinking or drugging spouse at home. The church can play a vital role in the recovery of both spouse and the addict.

More important, if the church is to be a force for change in the community, it must address the needs not just of those who attend church but of those who do not. Anyone in church who denies the need to help alcoholics and addicts is a destructive enabler. That irresponsible attitude needs to be replaced with care and concern, along with the action that produces change and hope. The ministry must be willing to reach beyond the church to help and for help. Addicts and alcoholics should be referred to treatment and supported once there. When the church decides to be aggressive and teach its members about addiction, it becomes a strong agent for prevention. The churches that go on to assist people in treatment provide the hope that has been lost for too long.

THE COUNSELORS

Therapists, counselors, and psychiatrists can unknowingly enable their clients by solving some problems, providing temporary relief, and dealing with the results of addiction rather than addiction itself. The uneducated counselor will attempt to relieve some of the symptoms of addiction. This delays recovery, and the addict is filled with false hopes that prevent long-term change. These professionals have immense potential to save thousands of lives. Statistics show that alcoholism affects one-third of all families in some way. Add drugs to that total and you find almost half the population plagued by addiction. If almost half of the general population has alcohol or drug problems, imagine what percentage of the people seeking help from a counselor are experiencing problems due to alcohol or drugs! It must approximate 70 or 80 percent, yet some counselors never consider alcohol or drugs. They just figure that if there is such a problem, it will subside when the psychological conflicts are resolved.

The counselor must probe into the drinking and drug history of the client. The client's family must be consulted to verify the information. If the counselor just assumes that everyone who walks in has an alcohol or drug problem, that counselor will be right more often than not. There should be regular referrals to treatment, where the counselor can follow the patient. A counselor alone is not powerful enough to stop the addiction process and start long-term recovery.

The counselor must refuse to accept the empty rationalizations of the addict that go with alcohol and drug abuse. The counselor must see through the rationalizations and into the reality of a life out of control. He or she must not get trapped by the reasoning that it can't be that bad if the patient retains the ability to control the drinking. Control has nothing to do with it. What is important are all the failed attempts to help. The counselor must act responsibly to be the person who finally initiates recovery for the alcoholic or addict. The rapport and trust built between therapist and client can be utilized to acquire the needed help for the addict and the addict's family.

If everyone in a community were determined to stop enabling the addict and the alcoholic, millions of lives would be saved every year. It is time that drug and alcohol problems become a priority in every city and town. The quick fix must be abandoned for the ultimate solution. Denial must be abandoned for the awareness that leads to corrective action. Each person must be committed to do his or her part to stop the misery and initiate recovery. When every element of society stops enabling, entire communities change. City by city and town by town, our world becomes a better place in which to live. We all can celebrate the new lives for alcoholics and addicts who would have remained sick, dying, and without help.

No matter what your role in your community, I urge you to act to change the place where you live. Become willing to do whatever it takes to rid your community of the destructive enabling that destroys lives, families, and even entire communities.

CHAPTER SIXTEEN

A SPECIAL MESSAGE TO MINISTERS

While treating alcoholics and drug addicts, my company did a research project to determine who the alcoholics and addicts talked to most frequently about their problem. When the results were tabulated, ministers emerged on top. Along the journey toward sobriety, those with chemical problems most frequently seek help from the clergy. For this reason, it is extremely important that everyone in the ministry have accurate information on which to build healthy attitudes. Currently, there are a lot of ministers who do not possess a loving or caring attitude toward the alcoholic. Although many seek advice or help from the clergy, they report rejection, judgmental attitudes, misinformation, and misdirection once they are face to face with a person in the ministry.

The following letter was sent to a group of ministers in Fort Worth, Texas. The purpose was to provide training and information to those who wanted it.

Dear Minister:

If you met Jim, he'd probably remind you of someone in your congregation.

Jim is intelligent, sensitive and responsible to his job, his loving family, and his God. But Jim has a serious disease, a disease you could help him conquer.

Jim is an alcoholic, but he won't admit it. He knows something is wrong and silently cries for help. Sometimes it seems hopeless. But for Jim and others like him, alcoholism can be treated. . . .

The response that most pathetically attracted my attention was this one:

Dear Administrator,

If Jim's problem is a disease, then alcoholic beverage companies are guilty of germ warfare. Jim is guilty of self-infliction of the germs.

When you people stop calling drunkenness a disease and spend as much time, money and effort to stop the sale of alcoholic beverages and start making responsible, intelligent, sensitive Jim pay for his misconduct instead of offering pity and justification to him, things will improve.

All Jims have a sickness *(but it is sin sickness).*

That response represents an attitude that hurts rather than helps alcoholics and addicts.

Can you imagine the anger and resentment behind the words of the writer? Can you imagine what a meeting would be like between this pastor and someone who had sought him out for help? What is so sad is that this letter genuinely represents the feelings of many people regarding the alcoholic and alcoholism. This is not just an isolated case of an angry preacher who is ignorant about the problem. Because this attitude is so common, I felt it would be helpful to look at the facts and attitudes that counter the pastor's approach to solving the problem.

First of all, this minister has a problem with labeling alcoholism as a disease. He only thinks of diseases as medical problems caused by germs. But a disease caused by spreading a germ is only one type of disease, a contagious disease. There are other types, such as hereditary diseases, which are not caused by passing a germ from one person to another. The disease is passsed through the genes of the parent to the child. Heart disease has proved to have a strong hereditary component; no germ causes a heart attack. Another type of disease that does not occur due to a germ is a developmental disease; hypertension is something many are not born with but develop through smoking, stress, poor diet, and lack of exercise. And of course, many problems are both developmental and hereditary. Diabetes, caused from genetic predisposition, develops over time with no germ as a factor. To discuss diseases intelligently, it is important to remember that they are not all caused by germs.

The minister also makes a mistake of equating drunkenness with alcoholism. He is saying that drunkenness is no disease; it is a sin. Well, I completely and thoroughly agree. I believe that anything irresponsible is sin. And I believe that whatever separates a person from God is a sin. Drunkenness is always irresponsible, and it always separates a person from God. Nothing good can come from drunkenness. Drunk people cause fatal traffic accidents and fatalities from guns and other violent acts. So when it comes to drunkenness, I agree with this pastor.

But drunkenness is not really what this pastor is speaking of. He has equated drunkenness with alcoholism. They are two completely different problems. Anyone who drinks can get drunk, but not everyone can become an alcoholic. And some alcoholics have a tolerance so high that they are never drunk. The drunkenness happens in the later stages, when the tolerance drops and the effect of the alcohol becomes unpredictable. The Bible quite clearly pronounces the evils of drunkenness; it is silent on alcoholism and addiction. I know of no one in the field of alcoholism or addiction who thinks that drunkenness is a disease. Drunkenness is always a very poor choice.

The pastor is also at odds with what he thinks the word disease does for Jim. He is afraid that it provides justification for the problem. Nothing could be further from the truth. Disease merely correctly labels the symptoms and problems that combine to form alcoholism, but no responsibility is removed. Anyone with pneumonia must accept responsibility to get the rest and nourishment needed to get well. No one can say that, since I have pneumonia, I am free to keep working and going out in the cold. Instead, once a person can accurately determine that pneumonia is the problem, then he or she can take precautions to ensure that the problem gets better instead of worse.

When diabetes is accurately diagnosed, the diabetic has hope. Medication and diet can be altered so that the symptoms of the disease do not occur. But a diabetic, knowing that diabetes is a disease, cannot just randomly eat sugar at will or act in a way that disregards the need for a change in life-style and diet. It is the same with the alcoholic. Labeling alcoholism as a disease does not free a person from the responsibility of getting well, but rather makes possible the progression toward getting well. Accepting the disease concept allows the alcoholic to accept treatment for the disease. That treatment must involve complete abstinence from alcohol. If a person does not believe alcoholism is a disease, use will probably continue. But among the various modalities of treatment comes one strong priority, complete abstinence.

The author of the letter is also very concerned that Jim pay for his misconduct rather than receive pity for it. Herein lies a central problem for many people. They are more concerned that justice be done than that help be obtained. The alcoholic is not short on guilt and shame, but guilt and shame do not produce recovery. They cause even more isolation and alienation. The alcoholic needs motivation to change. This motivation comes from corrective action taken by those close to the alcoholic. It does not come from pity, and it does not come from a judgmental or punitive attitude.

My desire for the alcoholic is not for more guilt, shame, and remorse, but for the alcoholic to change. That is not likely to happen when the alcoholic meets condemnation rather than caring confrontation. Help the alcoholic to find hope in recovery and there will be plenty of time—a lifetime—to make amends for a wasted past. The best way to make amends is by living sober one day at a time and accepting responsibility for resolving all the problems associated with drinking.

Numerous Christians, ministers, and professionals share my views about alcoholism. One of the best articles on the subject is found in the August 5, 1983 edition of *Christianity Today*. Barbara R. Thompson, in an article entitled ''Alcoholism: Even the Church Is Hurting,'' interviews Dr. Anderson Spickard, Jr., director of general internal medicine and a professor of medicine at Vanderbilt University Medical Center, as well as a practicing physician. He is also a Christian. In the interview he makes many points that I believe reflect truth and wisdom about alcoholism.

He believes that most are not aware of the extent of the problem in our churches. ''I think it is safe to assume that alcoholism and other forms of chemical dependency are playing a much larger role than we commonly believe.

"Also, there must be thousands, perhaps millions, of people who experienced the saving grace of Jesus as children or adolescents and have since dropped out of church because of their alcoholism. These people constitute a subclass of absolute despair within the body of Christ."

The fact that a Christian could become an alcoholic flies in the face of old beliefs of some rigid ministers. Viewing drinking as sin, they can in no way accept that a saved person can also be an alcoholic. But no one is immune. There are those who do not view drinking as wrong and innocently drink with no knowledge of the long-term outcome. They may find themselves in the middle of a tremendous drinking problem without ever perceiving its development.

When asked how a Christian can become an alcoholic, Dr. Spickard replied:

The same way it happens for anyone else. There are many factors, but two are the most pronounced: a genetic predisposition toward alcoholism and chronic, sustained drinking.

It is increasingly clear that there is an inherited physical susceptibility to alcoholism. A recent study from Sweden, where adoption records are well kept, shows that sons of alcoholic fathers placed at birth in nonalcoholic families have a nine-to-one chance of becoming alcoholics over adopted children born to nonalcoholic parents. This is an extraordinary statistic.

To the question, "Is there an alcoholic personality?" he responded,

No. Many studies have been done trying to establish a connection between certain kinds of personalities and alcoholism, but there is no evidence that one character type is more vulnerable than another. Anyone can become an alcoholic—even clergymen, and especially doctors.

In addressing the issue of drunkenness and alcoholism, Dr. Spickard explained well the difference:

Men and women who are merely abusing alcohol are still in control of their own will, and, unlike the alcoholic, they can usually quit whenever they choose. Perhaps a church member gets drunk at a New Year's Eve party, has an accident, and gets a Driving While Intoxicated citation. His family gets angry at him, he is socially embarrassed, and he promises never to drink again. That is the end of the problem.

This kind of alcohol abuse, while it may not lead to serious consequences, is addressed very pointedly in the Scriptures. Both Jesus and Paul warn us repeatedly that drunkards will not inherit the kingdom of God (Luke 21:34, I Cor. 6:10, Gal. 5:21). It's not hard to figure out why they speak so strongly: alcohol abuse is involved in most murders, most assaults, most child abuse cases, most traffic fatalities—the list is endless. We do ourselves and our entire society a great disservice when we laugh at drunkenness or treat it lightly.

The alcoholic, on the other hand, is one whose will has been captured by alcohol, who quite literally cannot stop drinking. He or she is in the grip of a progressive and complete destruction of his physical, mental, and spiritual being.

In response to the statement that some Christians see the disease concept as a behavioristic ploy and a humanistic interpretation of sin that denies the alcoholic's responsibility for his or her behavior, Dr. Spickard replied:

Alcohol abuse—drunkenness—is a sin. The Scripture is clear on this point. But once a person is an alcoholic, once he has allowed his will to be captured by alcohol through abuse, he is sick. He can no longer help himself. To tell an alcoholic to shape up and stop drinking is like telling a man who has just jumped out of a nine-story building to fall only three floors. It just isn't going to happen.

If we defined alcoholism as a physical disease, without a spiritual dimension, that might be humanism. There are many doctors and scientists looking for a physical cure for alcoholism. In my opinion, they won't find it. A person can have a physical illness, like cancer or tuberculosis, and still be perfectly fine emotionally and spiritually. No one can have alcoholism without being completely down the tubes physically, mentally, and spiritually. He will not get well until he is treated in all three areas. To insist upon this fact is not humanism; it is a holistic understanding of the patient.

The point is to get the alcoholic out of the arena of social moralizing and into the hands of people who can help him. The common perception of alcoholics is that they are hopeless cases. Yet 60 to 70 percent of all alcoholics who enter treatment programs recover.

Why does alcohol have such a devastating effect on the spiritual lives of heavy drinkers?

Alcohol is a mood-altering drug that directly affects the part of our brain that controls inhibitions. We all have built-in prohibitions against certain kinds of behavior. When these restraints are lowered through the use of alcohol, we find it much easier to violate our own moral standards.

A man with perfectly fine family values might drink too much, become euphoric, and climb into bed with his secretary. When the alcohol wears off, he is left with deep feelings of guilt and shame—and maybe a case of herpes. If the sin goes unconfessed, the feelings are suppressed, but the memory is still very much alive. The memory continually chips away at the man's already damaged moral life.

Put another way, if you accept the fact that drunkenness is a sin, which I do, then heavy drinking is just one more way to quench the Spirit. God has put His light within us, and it has the potential to burn as brightly as Jesus Himself. Sin darkens this light, and the drunkenness is as dark as anything there is in the world.''

On the church's response to alcoholism, Dr. Spickard explained:

The church should be in the forefront of efforts to help alcoholics because alcoholism has a pronounced spiritual dimension. Unfortunately, the church reflects the attitudes of society as a whole and looks at alcoholics as weak-willed and hopeless. Even well-meaning Christians tend to beat alcoholics over the head with a Bible, warning them to repent of their sin, and telling them not to come back to church until they can stop drinking. The alcoholic, no matter how sorry he feels, cannot stop—and he won't be back.

Many church members successfully conceal their alcoholism for years. They go to their pastors complaining of family or personal difficulties, but the root of their problem is never recognized and confronted. As their alcoholism progresses, these people drop out of church altogether. They can no longer afford the mental anguish that comes from rubbing shoulders with people they perceive as evangelical. The Christian alcoholic becomes convinced that he has lost his salvation and he doesn't darken the door of a church again. In this way he is effectively cut off from the people who should be most qualified to help him.

Lastly, Dr. Spickard addressed the concern of many evangelical Christians over the "vague spirituality" of Alcoholics Anonymous and the emphasis on a "higher power" and "God as we understand Him."

I know there are some evangelicals who believe that the only bona fide recovery programs are those that name the name of Jesus. From my viewpoint as a physician, this is short-sighted and prevents many people from getting the help they need. Because of their concentration on God as a "higher power," Alcoholics Anonymous has helped thousands of alcoholics from all religious persuasions, and Christian alcoholics have no trouble understanding this "higher power" as Jesus Christ.

In my own experience, with few exceptions, a person must first be sober before he can hear the gospel. I have a friend, a born-again surgeon and an alcoholic, who refused to go to Alcoholics Anonymous. He tried to get sober by going to Bible studies and prayer meetings, primarily because he didn't want to admit he was a drunk just like everyone else. He never could stop drinking. Finally, he humbled himself, admitted that he was powerless over his addiction, and went through the twelve steps of Alcoholics Anonymous. Today he is back at the Bible studies and prayer meetings and faithfully serving God.

When I read this article back in 1983, I was thrilled to see such a balanced approach published in a Christian magazine. I know its contents offended some at the time, as they do today, but it is full of truth and wisdom. I thank Barbara Thompson and Dr. Anderson Spickard, Jr., for this fine article that points to understanding and hope for the alcoholic.

There are those who simply refuse to address the problem of alcohol aand drugs within the church. Denial is the greatest factor in the reluctance to act. Many would say, "My church is different!" or "There is no alcoholism in our congregation," or "We don't even believe in drinking." But no church exists that does not experience the problem to some degree.

There may be no one who attends services in your church on Sunday who has an alcohol problem. But consider how many no longer go because drinking became such a problem. There are probably those who once attended regularly and now go somewhere else or not at all because they could no longer conceal the alcoholism. They fled before they were found out and condemned. There is a chance that they felt either no one cared or no one understood the problem.

It is also a strong possibility that some people show up in church alone because a spouse is either drinking or recovering from a drinking binge. It is common to see the silent "widows," whose marriage has died due to alcohol or drugs. They faithfully attend alone, praying that God will help. Without direction on how to intervene, they are faced with a life of despair. They need encouragement and direction on how to motivate the alcoholic or addict to obtain treatment. Preaching on the evils of alcoholism may prevent some from drinking, but it won't help those who are not there to hear because alcohol and drugs have destroyed their spiritual lives. To them the church represents guilt, condemnation, and rejection. They will stay away rather than be beaten up emotionally by those who do not seem to understand.

And although a congregation may be empty of heavy drinkers on Sunday morning, it is strongly possible that many there have parents with severe drinking problems. It is not uncommon for people whose parents had drinking problems to seek out a denomination where drinking is condemned. These people may possess years of hurt and bitterness masked by their Sunday morning best. Behind their stiff smiles and stiff clothing may be wounds of hurt and shame. These feelings can be resolved, but the issue of family alcoholism must be discussed if they are to be freed from the past.

Another consideration for any pastor not seeing alcohol and drugs as a problem is the kids in the church. Every church with teenagers who attend should address alcohol and drugs. Every day our kids, even elementary school kids, face pressure to drink and drug. Just saying "Don't do it!" is never enough. There must be a presentation of alternatives from an attitude of caring and understanding. The church is the institution that can do what parents and schools have often failed to do in the area of alcohol and drug abuse prevention. For a church to not help its kids make the right decision about alcohol and drugs is irresponsible. The uneasiness caused by addressing the topic is no excuse to ignore it.

Lastly, anyone denying the need for the church to take action should consider the role of the church in the community. The church is not to be an isolated band of "holy huddlers" who have no impact on the community. The church is to be a force for positive change and community reform. Every community has an alcohol and drug problem. It cannot simply be legislated away. For too long the church has allowed schools and government agencies to be the ones to work with those who have chemical abuse problems but that must stop. The church has the resources and the motivation to help people with alcohol and drug problems in the community. And as these people are assisted, they are attracted to the church, not repelled from it. When the church gets busy helping people with alcohol and drug problems, communities get better.

No church is immune from drug and alcohol problems, just as no community is immune from them. But what can a church do if it is motivated to help but doesn't know exactly what to do? Many things can become part of a strategy. But before examining those, it is important to address the drinking issue. There is nothing wrong with preaching against drinking or drugs, but sermons must not be considered the entire solution. Statistics show that at least 97 percent of all high school seniors have consumed alcohol. If someone tells seniors the best prevention is to never take the first drink, then only 3 percent of the audience has any chance of benefiting from the presentation. The drinking issue is an important one to deal with. It is helpful to assist people in considering the "rightness" or "wrongness" of drinking, but it is more important, since so many make the decision to drink, that attention be focused on how to help those who made the choice and found the experience to be anything but pleasurable. When a church decides to forsake a judgmental role and reach out to those who drink and drug, the church, the community, and especially the alcoholics and addicts benefit greatly.

OPTIONS FOR THE CHURCH

I was asked to give a six-week course on alcohol and drugs for the church I was attending in Newport Beach. To promote the class, the pastor interviewed me in front of the church. When I spoke to the congregation for the first time, I told them that our church, and many churches, had a problem with alcohol and drugs. I said that at least one-third of all families report a problem with alcohol. I said that it is quite possible that the person sitting next to you could be an alcoholic. I then invited each person to look to the left and right to see if they could determine whether the person sitting next to them was an alcoholic. The second I said this, there was giggling and laughter as the people looked at each other. Then I changed the crowd's mood. I said that from the laughter it was obvious that an attitude problem existed within the church. I asked them to consider what had just transpired.

What had happened was that the whole congregation had laughed at the prospect of being seated next to an alcoholic, someone with a fatal and chronic disease. I asked them to consider another scenario. I asked them to think of their reaction if I had said my topic was not alcoholism, but instead, cancer. It would certainly not have aroused laughter, but sadness and compassion. There would have been a sincere attempt to comfort the person who was struggling with cancer. There would have been silence, not laughter.

My fellow church members certainly got the point. As a result, over two hundred people have been trained in the area of alcoholism and drug addiction. In the twelve months that followed, at least fifty people from the church entered treatment, and hundreds of lives have been changed. The church even collected special offerings to fund the treatment of some of its members. Either directly or indirectly, almost everyone had a part in the recovery of churchgoers who had been ignored. Any church can have the same experience. Every congregation has those in need of guidance and direction. When the church makes up its mind to help, there are many who will be helped. The following ideas can be implemented by any church dedicated to changing the lives of alcoholics and drug addicts. But to be effective, alcohol problems must not be treated as if they were a rash among the congregation. Alcoholism must be considered a problem in need of major surgery. Far below the surface rests the real severity of the problem. Correct action will involve whatever it takes to uncover the problem and assist those in need of help.

1. The place to begin to help people is from the pulpit. It is the only way to reach out to the one-third of your families who have been affected by alcoholism. What problem deserves more attention than this one? It has become a national scourge. Invite knowledgeable speakers at least twice a year to address the problem. Include the issue in sermons along the way during the year. It is important to consider the focus of the message. Any alcoholic or drug addict is aware of how bad the problem is, but he or she is not aware of how much hope is available. Counterbalancing any message on the evils of alcoholism must be a presentation of the hope to be found in recovery. In addition, those families who are going through the problem must be made aware that the preacher and the entire church care about the alcoholic and the addict. The amount of caring is far more valuable to those families than the amount of knowledge possessed by the pastor. The pulpit is the place to begin. When messages about "sorry alcoholics" are replaced with hope for recovery, people will seek out the minister to obtain help and start over.

2. Small group studies are important to supplement what is taught from the pulpit. Whether it is a church study course or a

mini-church study, the small group is where specific issues can be handled. When the leaders of these groups feel incompetent to handle all of the issues raised, it is easy to acquire chemical dependency experts who will serve as a resource. Many Scriptures can be used to reinforce the need for reaching out to the alcoholic and the alcoholic's family. These biblical passages can form the basis of a study of the lives of alcoholics, addicts, and their families. It can also lead to answers for those in the midst of a chemical crisis at home.

3. In addition to training for everyone, there should be an advanced training course. Out of this course will come many volunteers who will intervene for the church in the lives of those with alcohol and drug problems. These people can form a task force that is available twenty-four hours a day to help anyone who has a problem. They may also form recovery support groups for those who want long-term support from the church. This core of committed counselors can be an invaluable resource to the church and facilitate the recovery of both active and inactive church members.

4. Whether they are called bishops, elders, or deacons, the leadership of the church needs this special training. Without it, the needs of the church members cannot and will not be met. Raising the awareness of the church leadership allows alcoholics and addicts to receive help, no matter what the surface problem is. When elders, deacons, and bishops are trained, they are better able to uncover the fact that alcohol and drugs are the real source of difficulty and direct the person to the appropriate resource.

5. Some churches employ a full-time intervention counselor who does nothing but work with chemical abuse problems. This person conducts classes and leads families through the intervention process. When this service is provided within the church, it allows for closer follow-up of recovery by the church. It can be expanded to help intervene in the lives of those with other problems, such as eating, sex, and gambling. Christ was the original interventionist. When He lashed out at the money changers in the temple, He was essentially intervening in their lives. He was no longer willing for them to live as they had been living. An interventionist directs people away from destruction and toward a better life.

6. For the Christian churches, AA meetings, with Christ as a higher power, can provide needed balance for recovery. Having AA meetings within the church allows people to feel safe to confront the problem. An indirect stamp of approval is placed on obtaining help. Barring recovery groups such as AA from the church does just the opposite. It allows alcoholics and addicts to feel further rejection and compels them to go outside the church for help.

7. Telephone counselors, available twenty-four hours a day, can be a valuable resource for those who want help. Calling anonymously can be a first step toward complete recovery. Phones do not have to be staffed; phone counselors just need to be available when someone does call. It is surprising how many people want to be a part of a telephone counseling ministry.

8. As people begin to recover within the church, a group of people usually develops who are willing to go into homes and personally visit those who call for help. After years of isolation and alienation, this initial visit can establish the fact that people care. With training, these visitors can be a valuable extension to those who handle crises over the phone. The church is no stranger to home visitation; it should not neglect this unique opportunity.

9. Some people are too threatened even to call for help, but they will pick up literature that addresses the problem. Every sect, denomination, and religion should produce written materials on alcohol and drugs that present the facts in accordance with that group's dogma or theology—that is, of course, if the philosophy is in accordance with principles that help rather than hurt. People are always asking, "Do you have something I could read on alcohol and drugs?" It is very helpful to have those resource materials available.

10. One of the areas that must be addressed by the church is the pressure for kids to use drugs and alcohol. Bring someone in to discuss drinking and drugs with them as early as elementary school. The church can be the first to introduce positive alternatives to drugs and alcohol. But waiting until junior high is much too late; our children are confronted with alcohol and drugs as early as kindergarten. The church should not remain silent. Drug and alcohol education from the church

can turn many temptations into opportunities for self-discipline.

11. Training must not be limited to the children and teenagers. Parents need help in dealing with this very complex issue. The tendency for most parents today is to claim that it could never happen to their kids. They are uncomfortable in talking about the topic, so they procrastinate, hoping that someone else will handle the problem; but the problem must be handled by the parents. Discussions need to focus on accurate information and the consequences of irresponsible drinking and drug use. The only solid counter to negative peer pressure is positive family reinforcement. The best positive reinforcement is an open forum where drugs and alcohol can be discussed. The church can train parents to feel competent in handling these issues.

12. Special groups, men's and women's, need to realize the need for education on alcohol and drugs and bring in speakers for specific instruction and training. The next step is for the training to be expanded into neighborhoods and businesses of those in the special church groups. Infiltration into neighborhoods and businesses with good alcohol and drug information and methods of helping expands the role of the church. The church becomes the strong agent of change, not concerned just with those who show up on Sundays but also with those who might never enter the church doors.

13. The last, and I believe most important, alternative for the church is to itself provide counseling and therapeutic support. Group therapy and recovery support groups directed by qualified leaders are very effective in meeting people's needs. If people come to attend the recovery groups, they may stay and attend church, so the process is also a tool for church growth. Even more important, it is a means by which the church can demonstrate its concern. It is a visible means of welcoming the alcoholic in rather than keeping him or her out.

These are but a few examples of what a church can do to reach out and help alcoholics. Merely to sit back and pray is irresponsible. Action must accompany the prayer. A concept reflected in a story I heard when I was young is relevant here. Two little girls on their way to school heard the bell ring. They had been tardy twice before and would be expelled if they were late one more time. One little girl said, "Let's climb down into the ditch and pray." The other little girl said, "I think we should pray while we run."

Be the leader to reach out to alcoholics. Pray for alcoholics and addicts while you run to help them find hope.

Addiction Tapes

The material presented here is available on cassette tape. The four tapes, recorded by Stephen Arterburn are designed to share with someone who might have an addiction problem or a co-dependent family member. The cost for the set is $29.95, including postage and handling. To obtain a set send $29.95 to:

The Addiction Tapes
Outreach Ministries
Box 4947
Laguna Beach, CA 92652

For information on seminars and lectures by Stephen Arterburn, phone (714) 494-8383.

Additional Help

If you or someone in your family needs help with an addiction problem, phone New Life Treatment Centers at 1-800-227-LIFE.

Bibliography

Alcohol Abuse in America. The Gallup Organization, conducted for CareUnit Hospital Program. Princeton, New Jersey, November 1982.

Alcohol and Health. First Special Report to the U.S. Congress, DHEW Publication No. (HSM) 72-9099. Washington, D.C.: U.S. Government Printing Office, 1971.

Alcoholics Anonymous. New York City: Alcoholics Anonymous World Services, 1976.

Alcoholism Report. March 17, 1983.

Bacon, M. K. "Cross-cultural Studies of Drinking." *Alcoholism, Progress in Research and Treatment*. P. G. Bourne & R. Fox (Eds.). New York: Academic Press, 1973.

Bohman, M.; Sigvardsson, S.; Cloninger, C. "Maternal Inheritance of Alcohol Abuse—Cross Fostering Analysis of Adopted Women." *Archives of General Psychiatry*, vol. 38, September 1981.

Bohman, Michael. "Some Genetic Aspects of Alcoholism and Criminality." *Archives of General Psychiatry*, vol. 38, September 1981.

Cadoret, R. J.; Cain, C. A.; Grove, W. M. "Development of Alcoholism in Adoptees Raised Apart from Biological Relatives." *Archives of General Psychiatry*, vol. 37 (May 1980).

Cadoret, R. J., and Gath, A. "Inheritance of Alcoholism in Adoptees." *British Journal of Psychiatry* (1978).

Castro, Janice. "Buried in a Tropical Snowstorm." *Time* (March 17, 1986).

Cloninger, C. R.; Christiansen, K. O.; Reich, T.; Gottesman, I. I. "Implications of Sex Differences in the Prevalences of Antisocial Personality, Alcoholism, and Criminality for Familial Transmission." *Archives of General Psychiatry*, vol. 35, August 1978.

Cloninger, C. R.; Bohman, M.; Sigvardsson, S. "Inheritance of Alcohol Abuse Cross-Fostering Analysis of Adopted Men." *Archives of General Psychiatry*, vol. 38 (August 1981).

"Cocaine Babies: Hooked at Birth." *Newsweek* (July 18, 1986).

"Cocaine, the Deadliest." *Alcoholism and Addiction Magazine* (February, 1986).

"Crack and Crime." *Newsweek* (June 16, 1986).

El-Guebaly, N., and Offord, D. R. "The Offspring of Alcoholics: A Critical Review." *The American Journal of Psychiatry*, vol. 134:4 (April 1977).

"Ethanol Ingestion: Differences in Blood Acetaldehyde Concentrations in Relatives of Alcoholics and Controls." *Science*, vol. 203 (January 5, 1979).

Frances, R. J.; Timm, S.; Bucky, S. "Studies of Familial and Nonfamilial Alcoholism." *Archives of General Psychiatry*, vol. 37 (May 1980).

"Genetic Factors in Alcoholism." *Center for Alcohol Studies*, vol. 1, no. 1 (September 1980) Chapel Hill, North Carolina.

Gleaton, T. J., and Gowen, S. "The Adolescent Drug Epidemic and Chronic Young Adult Patient: Is There a Link?" *Psychiatry Letter*, vol. III (February 1985).

Gold, Mark S. *800-COCAINE*. New York: Bantam, 1984.

Goodwin, D. W. "Alcoholism and Heredity." *Archives of General Psychiatry*, vol. 36 (January 1979).

Goodwin, D. W. "Genetic Components of Alcoholism." *Annual Review of Medicine*, vol. 32 (1981).

Goodwin, D. W. "Is Alcoholism Hereditary?" *Archives of General Psychiatry*, vol. 25 (December 1971).

Goodwin, D. W.; Powell, B.; Stern, J. "Behavioral Tolerance to Alcohol in Moderate Drinkers." *American Journal of Psychiatry*, vol. 127:12 (June 1971).

Goodwin, D. W.; Schulsinger, F.; Hermansen, L.; Guze, S. B.; Winokur, G. "Alcohol Problems in Adoptees Raised Apart from Alcoholic Biological Parents." *Archives of General Psychiatry*, vol. 28 (February 1973).

Goodwin, D. W.; Schulsinger, F.; Knop, J.; Mednick, S.; Guze, S. "Alcoholism and Depression in Adopted-out Daughters of Alcoholics." *Archives of General Psychiatry*, vol. 34 (July 1977).

Goodwin, D. W.; Schulsinger, F.; Knop, J.; Mednick, S.; Guze, S. B. "Psychopathology in Adopted and Nonadopted Daughters of Alcoholics." *Archives of General Psychiatry*, vol. 34 (September 1977).

Goodwin, D. W.; Schulsinger, F.; Moller, N.; Hermansen, L.; Winokur, G.; Guze, S. B. "Drinking Problems in Adopted and Nonadopted Sons of Alcoholics." *Archives of General Psychiatry*, vol. 31 (August 31, 1974).

Goodwin, D. W. "The Genetics of Alcoholism." *Substance and Alcohol Actions/Misuse*, 1980.

"Groups Found to Differ in Reaction to Alcohol." *NIAAA Information and Feature Service* (December 31, 1981).

Jellinek, E. M. *The Disease Concept of Alcoholism*. New Haven, Connecticut: College and University Press Services, 1960.

Johnson, N. *NIAAA Information and Feature Service*, no. 99 (August 30, 1982).

Johnson, E., Nilsson, T. "Alkohol-Konsumption Ho s Monozygota och Dizygota Tvillangar." *Nord. Hyg. Tidskr*, vol. 49:21, 1968.

Kaij, Lennart, and Dock, J. "Grandsons of Alcoholics." *Archives of General Psychiatry*, vol. 32 (November 1975).

Kerr, Peter. "New Form of Cocaine Brings Renewed Concern Over Drugs." *Orange County Register*, August 10, 1986.

"Kids and Cocaine." *Newsweek* (March 17, 1986).

Kolata, Gina. "Study Finds Difference In Cells of Alcoholics." *New York Times*, Living Arts Section, Thursday, September 15, 1988.

Kurtz, E. "Why A. A. Works. The Intellectual Significance of Alcoholics Anonymous." *Journal of Studies on Alcohol*, vol. 43, 1982.

Landsbaum, Mark. "County's Affluent Attracts Growing Cocaine Trade." *Los Angeles Times*, January 26, 1986.

Layden, T. A., and Smith, J. W. "Nonmetric Pattern Analysis of Behavioral and Biological Disease Symptoms in Alcoholism." *Archives of General Psychiatry*, vol. 25 (February 1973).

Lamar Jr., Jacob. "Crack." *Time* (June 2, 1986).

Lemere, F. "The Nature and Significance of Brain Damage from Alcoholism." *American Journal of Psychiatry*, vol. 113, 1956.

Lipscomb, T. R.; Carpenter, J. A.; Nathan, P. E. "Static Ataxia: A Predictor of Alcoholism?" *British Journal of Addiction*, vol. 74, 1979.

Lipscomb, T. R., and Nathan, P. E. "Blood Alcohol Level Discrimination—The Effects of Family History on Alcoholism, Drinking Pattern and Tolerance." *Archives of General Psychiatry*, vol. 37 (May 1980).

Los Angeles Times, December 1, 1985.

Ludwig, A. M., and Wikler, A. "Craving and Relapse to Drink." *Quarterly Journal of Studies on Alcoholism*, vol. 35, 1974.

Luks, Allan. "The 'Sober Up' Pill: A Possible Cure for Drunkenness." *The Futurist* (October 1981).

Martz, Larry et al. "Trying to Say No." *Newsweek* (August 11, 1986).

Mello, Nancy K. "Etiological Theories of Alcoholism." *Advances in Alcoholism*, vol. II (June 1981).

Mello, N. K., and Mendelson, J. H. "Alcohol and Human Behavior," in L. L. Iverson, S. D. Iverson & S. H. Snyder (Eds.). *Handbook of Psychopharmacology. Drugs of Abuse*, vol. 12, New York: Plenum Publishing, 1978.

Mendelson, J. H.; La Dou, J.; Solomon, P. "Experimentally Induced Chronic Intoxication and Withdrawal in Alcoholics: III Psychiatric

Findings." *Quarterly Journal of Studies on Alcoholism*, supplement 2, 1964.

Milam, James R. & Ketcham, Katherine. *Under the Influence*. Seattle: Madronna Publishers, 1981.

"New York City Being Swamped by Crack." *Los Angeles Times*, August 1, 1986.

Ohlms, David L. *The Disease Concept of Alcoholism*. Belleville, Illinois: Gary Whiteaker Company, 1983.

Partanen, J., Brunn, K., Markanen, T. "Inheritance of Drinking Behavior: A Study of Intelligence, Personality & Use of Alcohol of Adult Twins." *Alcohol Research in Northern Countries*, Helsinki Finnish Foundation for Alcohol Studies, 1966.

Propping, P.; Kruger, J.; Mack, N. "Genetic Disposition to Alcoholism. An EEG Study in Alcoholics and Their Relatives." *Human Genetics*, vol. 59, 1981.

Robins, L. N.; Bates, W. M.; O'Neal, P. "Adult Drinking Patterns of Former Problem Children." *Society, Culture and Drinking Patterns*. New York: John Wiley & Sons, Inc., 1962.

Rosett, H. L. "Clinical Pharmacology of the Fetal Alcohol Syndrome." *Biochemistry & Pharmacology of Ethanol*. New York: Plenum Press, Inc., 1979.

Saunders, J. B. "Alcoholism: New Evidence for a Genetic Contribution." *British Medical Journal*, vol. 284.

Schuckit, Mark A.; Goodwin, Donald A.; Winokur, George. "A Study of Alcoholism in Half Siblings." *American Journal of Psychiatry*, vol. 128 (March 1972).

Schuckit, M., and Vidamantas, R. "Ethanol Ingestion: Differences in Blood Acetaldehyde Concentrations in Relatives of Alcoholics and Controls." *Science*, vol. 203 (January 5, 1979).

This World, November 3, 1985.

Time Magazine, December 23, 1985.

USA Today, December 22, 1985.

USA Today, December 27, 1985.

USA Today, November 8, 1985.

USA Today, October 25, 1985.

USA Today, October 10, 1985.

U.S. Journal, November 1985.

U.S. News & World Report, November 18, 1985.

Valliant, G. E. *Adolf Meyer Was Right: Dynamic Psychiatry Needs the Life Chart*. Streker Monograph Series #16, 1979.

Washton, Arnold M. "Cocaine Abuse Treatment." *Psychiatry Letter*, vol. III (September 1985).

Washton, Arnold M. "Teen Use Increasing." *U.S. Journal of Alcohol and Drug Dependency*, October 1985.

Weiner, S.; Tamerij, J.; Steinglass, P.; Mendelson, J. "Familial Patterns in Chronic Alcoholism: A Study of a Father and Son During Experimental Intoxication." *American Journal of Psychiatry*, vol. 127 (June 1971).

"Wild Drunks and 'Sick' Alcoholics May Have Different Genes." *Medical World News*, August 2, 1982.

Wolf, Peter H. "Ethnic Differences in Alcohol Sensitivity." *Science*, vol. 175 (January 28, 1972).

Index

About the Author

STEPHEN F. ARTERBURN has been involved in the past twelve years with programs designed to motivate people with problems to take responsibility for their own recovery at counseling centers, psychiatric hospitals, and chemical dependency treatment centers. For nine years he worked for Comprehensive Care Corporation in a variety of management positions. From there he became President and Chief Executive Officer of Westworld Community Healthcare that developed drug and pain treatment centers across the country. In 1988 he founded a behavioral health care company called New Life Treatment Centers that treats psychiatric, alcohol and drug problems in a Christ-centered program. Mr. Arterburn received his bachelor's degree from Baylor University and his master's degree from North Texas State University. He is a nationally known speaker, author and coauthor of the following books: *Growing Up Addicted, How Will I Tell My Mother?*, *When Someone You Love Is Someone You Hate*, and *Drug-Proof Your Kids*. He and his wife Sandy live in Laguna Beach, California.